Take YOUR *Life* Back

*A compelling true story
about the pain and heartache
of childhood, teen, and adult obesity.*

HOW DOES OBESITY HAPPEN TO A CHILD TOO LITTLE TO REACH THE COOKIE JAR?

Lois Peres

Take Your Life Back

How does obesity happen to a child too little to reach the cookie jar?

If you would like to order more books, please contact us
www.youcantakeyourlifeback.org

Dedication

I offer this book as a gift of hope for those who have suffered or are suffering from obesity. There is an answer for you. To start with, know that God really does love you. Do not ever think He doesn't. You may be asking, "Why then am I in the state that I'm in if God loves me?" I answer this question and much more in the pages of this book. Read on, my friend, there are answers and hope.

Lois J. Peres

Table of Contents

Foreword by Pastor *Jeff Crume*

You *meet* a lot of people in a lifetime, but you really get to *know* very few of them. If you are fortunate, from those *few* you really get to know, you find a friend; a confidant, one who will make a lasting impact on your life – that's Lois.

I've known Lois Peres for almost fifteen years. I started out working for her in the phone ministry at Cottonwood Christian Center where we both attended church. Little did I know, that over the years, I would be so fortunate to develop a friendship and relationship with Lois, and her husband, Gerson, that would go on to have a profound impact on my life, my family, and my ministry.

Over the years, Lois has been "Mema" to my children, a friend to my wife and I, and my Associate Pastor. But above all, Lois has been my friend and confidant. Proverbs 18:24 says, *"there is a friend who sticks closer than a brother"* – that's Lois.

Through the years, Lois has been there by my side every step of the way. She has been a voice of encouragement, a voice of instruction and correction, constantly reminding me of who I am and what I can accomplish through Christ Jesus. Lois kept me going when I wanted to quit, picked me up when I fell down, and turned the other cheek when I would lash out at her in my early years of frustration and immaturity. She is truly a *friend who sticks closer than a brother.*

I'm honored to introduce Lois Peres to you and recommend her new book, *"Take Your Life Back."* If anyone can help you *take your life back*, it's Lois. What you are reading is not just a book; it's a living testimony, one that I've had the privilege of being an eyewitness to over the years of knowing Lois. Are you struggling with Obesity? This book is for you. Are you desperately trying to discover who you are and what you were put on this earth to do?

This book is for you. Are you searching for meaning in life? This book is for you.

Just a word of caution: don't allow yourself to just read this book and put it on the shelf. Discipline yourself to do what this book says to do; if you do, you too can *Take Your Life Back*! Go ahead, what are you waiting for? Get started today.

Jeff Crume, Pastor
Jeff Crume Ministries

Acknowledgements

The Love of God is without description. It is too awesome for words. I thank the Lord for His patience and endurance with me while writing this book. May it glorify Him alone.

I offer unending thanks to Gerson, my husband, without whose love and strong encouragement I could not have even started such an encounter. His dedication to me and to God is without measure. I am truly blessed and honored with such a gift as him.

I would like to give a special thanks and appreciation to someone that has stuck closer than a brother. Pastor Jeff Crume has not only been an encouragement, he has been a friend in the true sense of the word. He has kept me motivated, focused, challenged, and corrected.

He is by no means just a friend, but my pastor as well. His spiritual insight, as well as his practical knowledge of authoring books himself, has helped me greatly. Pastor Jeff has contributed tremendous time and effort into the design of the book cover, as well as input in the formatting of the entire book. Thank you for your investment in me, and all who will receive great help from the words of this book.

Lois J. Peres

I

The Great Weight Battle

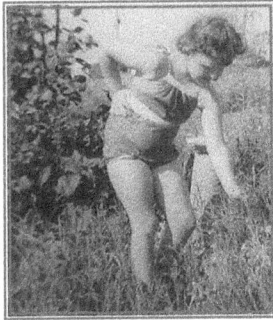

As far back as my memory will take me, I struggled with being overweight. At the age of five, I was already bigger than my older brother and weighed close to seventy pounds. They called it "baby fat," and thought it was cute. When does it stop being baby fat and start becoming a problem? When do we, as a parent or guardian, begin to be concerned that our child's baby fat is increasing? These are questions that every parent needs to answer.

At the young age of five, I had no concept of what being overweight or underweight meant, nor should I have. A five-year old eats what she/he is given. So, where does the problem lie? Most everyone knows it is the responsibility of the parent or guardian to monitor the food intake of a child. What happens when the caregiver has little or no knowledge of the proper way to feed a growing child?

We are experiencing a generation of childhood obesity like never before. *The Clinton Foundation* says that today, nearly 25 million children are overweight or obese. *The National Center for Chronic Disease Prevention and Health Promotion* tells us that in the past 30 years childhood obesity has tripled. We hear it every day on the news and on talk shows. The obesity rate is out of control. I was one of these children caught up in that rising rate of obesity. I will be sixty years of age this year and I was raised by very loving, but uninformed parents who thought food was an expression of love. They replaced the words, "I love you" with a big piece of chocolate cake with ice cream on top. At the time, I felt the love in that! But what happens when the love turns to weight and then to hate?

According to the stories I've heard, my parents never had enough to eat growing up. They lived in the days of the Depression, and it was a struggle to stay alive. This poverty-ridden life continued into the early days of their marriage. It was then passed on to us kids. Remembering back, as a child we ate a lot of rabbits, chicken, potatoes, and macaroni. We ate what was available. The problem began when my mother fried everything in lard, to make it taste better. She had no idea at the time just how unhealthy this way of cooking was. We were encouraged to eat all that was given on our plates, because of all the people who had nothing. Somehow that made sense to them. Things are quite different now days. Most people do have a choice what to eat, how to cook it properly, and what to feed their families.

I hear many mothers today saying that it is just too expensive to eat healthy. I disagree. Fruits and vegetables are just as cheap as macaroni and cheese. (I can hear some objecting right now with that statement.) Let's just think about this. I have found that it doesn't take any more to feed a family healthy food as opposed to high-calorie foods *if we stay within the right portion sizes.* The problem begins when we serve three or four servings at once. It cost more money and makes overweight families.

Many of us need to break some bad habits. If we really want to help our kids live long and strong, we must research portion sizes and explore different foods. Eating more live foods, such as different fruits, vegetables, nuts and grains is not any more expensive than eating high carbohydrate, high calorie foods. We can also start teaching our children at a young age to explore and enjoy a different variety of the things we are already eating. For instance, there are many different kinds of squash, onions and lettuce. They look different and taste different. Nuts are a fun thing to explore with kids. I can't even tell you how many different kinds there are. Have fun and try them all. We'll learn more about better choices in a future chapter.

"Experts tell us that we can either make or break a habit in 21 days."

൮

2

Killing With Kindness

In 1956, we moved from Wichita, Kansas to Bellflower, California. My father was offered a wonderful job with the fire department, at Rockwell International, in Downey, CA. and things were looking up. The money started coming in, and so did the food. I remember sitting down to the most wonderful seven-course meals you could imagine. My mom and dad were making up for lost time. We ate like there was no tomorrow. Friday night was my favorite time of the week. My parents, two brothers, John and Dennis, and I would pile into the car and be off to the market. We were so amazed at all the different foods. We wanted to try everything, and we did. Super-sized!

My parents didn't realize that they were beginning to unintentionally train us to continually overeat and make bad choices.

> *"The bigger I got, the more I ate; the more I ate, the more I wanted."*

Before we moved from Kansas, we children thought that rabbits and chickens were *it!* We only got to experience candy when we visited our rich aunt. I found out later she wasn't rich at all. They didn't have the expense of a family and could afford the luxuries of candies. My Aunt Elaine was a beautiful woman but she was very overweight. Now, *we* were the rich ones. It seemed like it, anyway. My parents introduced us to cake, pie, candy, ice cream, and cookies.

We had roast with potatoes and gravy, big biscuits with lots of jam, big salads—and don't forget desserts. We ate like kings every night of the week. You see, my parents thought they were being kind to us by showing their love through making sure we were full all the time. In reality, they were setting up a lifestyle of food addiction.

∽

3

They Didn't Know

All parents want the very best for their children, and my parents were no exception. They wanted us to have the things they never had. My dad would tell us heartbreaking stories about how he and his brother had to steal food for themselves and their sister. My dad was only about eight years old when his mother died. My grandfather Joe, was away most of the time. If they wanted to eat, they had to get food the only way they knew how.

My father even had food issues from a very young age. I am sure that not having enough to eat does unimaginable things to one's mind. He vowed that he would never go without food when he grew up. His sister and brothers made the same vow, and they ended up being very overweight adults. They all had overweight children as well—except for one. My Uncle Bud married a woman who practiced healthy eating. Their children were thin and healthy, unlike the children of the overweight siblings.

It all comes down to the choices we are taught to make. The good thing is, we can retrain ourselves and break free from old habits. If we can learn healthy choices and get used to eating sensibly when we're young, it will be much easier to keep on track as an adult and share our good habits with the future generations. Don't fall for the lie that you have to be rich to eat right—it's not true. In my case, having more money helped put weight on me. It takes more than money to eat well—we need to be wise enough to make good choices.

∽ 4 ∽

The "O" Word

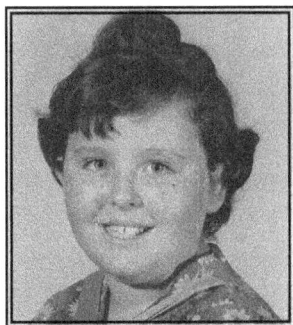

Over time, I began to gain weight like crazy. The weird thing was that my brothers didn't expand as fast as I did at the time. So what was this all about? Most of the time we ate the same things at the same time. I remember I was the one who cleared the table every night and ate the leftovers. That might account for it. By the age of nine I wasn't just fat anymore. I begin to show signs of the "O–word" manifesting itself: *obesity.* What was that? Was I going to die? I didn't even feel sick. After the doctor explained what it was, I wanted to die. My parents lowered my food intake for a while and assumed I would just grow out of it.

My advice to parents is to take these kind of reports seriously. Yes, some children might grow out of it, but what if your child does not? It becomes a battle that many times didn't need to be fought. My life was getting worse by minute. I didn't lose weight. The fact is, my parents got busy with *life stuff,* and forgot about watching my food intake most of the time.

As for me, I was already one of fattest kids in the entire school. I was called every fat name in the book. I remember crying a lot and my mother would say, "If you don't like being called names, then just quit eating." Somehow, being an overweight nine-year-old seemed to be my fault, and it was up to me fix it.

Well, as much as I hated being call "fat-so," and hearing the clever little song, "Fatty, fatty, two by four, can't get through the bathroom door, so she did it on the floor," I couldn't lose weight. I got bigger and bigger. By this time I was in the third grade and was close to 150 pounds. My heart goes out to all the little children today who are suffering as I did. My hope is that this book will help open the eyes of parents and caregivers alike. It's not easy to tell your child "No," where food is concerned, but in many cases, it's the right thing to do. It might make them mad at the time, but I promise you, they'll appreciate it later in life.

ॐ

~5~

School Days

School had always been like punishment to me. Even in the lower grades, kids learned to be very cruel. On the way to school, I would stop at a little market where I could buy candy with my lunch money. That bought me a friend for the day; otherwise, it was hard to get anyone to play with me. Being fat was like having a disease.

Lunch did not seem to be a problem. I would eat what kids left on their trays, which was usually a lot. In those days, the schools served a lot of things many of the kids didn't like. They would serve meatloaf, baked chicken, sweet potatoes, tuna casseroles and the likes. Carrots, mashed potatoes and corn were plentiful. Even then, the schools served very high carbohydrate meals. There was always plenty for me to eat. Today there are fast food vendors right inside the school. Kids can get burgers, fries, and pizza without leaving campus.

> *"Schools have become one of the biggest contributors to the childhood obesity epidemic in the United States."*

It appears that the current food regulations are not working.

Big-Mouthed Nurse

Now back to the trauma of the "fat schooldays." If you are a parent or guardian, please listen to me. Perhaps you will save your child from an enormous amount of pain. It is humiliating and stressful to always be picked last for any games. The other children knew that I wasn't very fast because of my weight and I got tired quickly. They anticipated a loss if they were to be stuck with me on their team. Many times the teacher would have to force them to play with me.

One of the worst parts of the school year was the day we would all go to the nurse to be weighed. On that day, the nurse would call out my weight in front of everyone. Talk about wanting to die. It seemed like no one considered my feelings. My teachers, and family would just tell me to *"lose weight."* How could adults be so blind? I would like to know.

Parents, please don't get so busy with your own issues that you forget your children's health and well-being. Yes, it is very important to make money so you can give your children the finer things in life, but if they are too sick to enjoy them, what have you gained?

Remember, people can be very cruel; even teachers, friends, and family members can say things that could devastate and scar a child forever. You can change the outcome of your child's future

~

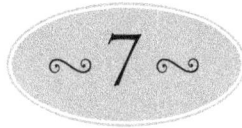

Fat Cells

Medical science tells us that the average person has twenty-five to thirty-five billion fat cells. Fat cells expand or contract as we gain or lose weight. The bad thing is they never go away. Our fat cells are always demanding more. As we grow, fat cells become "food beggars." The more they beg, the more we feed them; the more we feed them, the more they grow; the more they grow; the more we increase in weight and size.

There are two critical times in our life when fat cells develop the most. The first time is when a child is around two years of age. An alarming number of two-year olds today are overweight. Some are even reaching weights of 150 pounds.

The second time fat cells develop the most is during adolescence. Without proper supervision, especially in the pre-teen years, a child can be set up for a lifetime of sickness and suffering. These are not the only times fat cells are developed, but they are the most critical times of fat cell development.

We have been deceived into thinking that it is just baby fat. I have news for you: fat is fat, whether you are two or twenty-two. So, next time you are thinking about giving your two-year old a cupcake and chips for a smack, just because he or she asks for one, give them an apple instead. As parents and grandparents, we need to wise up. There is so much information available about nutrition. I know you love your kids just as I love mine. You want to help them have a better childhood. Do not let this go. It could be a matter of life or death.

⤳

~ 8 ~

Sabotaging Our Kids

My heart breaks for the kids I see today that are so overweight. I know the pain and humiliation these kids must be going through. I want to get a hold of them and tell them that it is not their fault. Then whose responsibility is it for the rise in childhood obesity? I think we all know the answer to this question: most likely it's mom and dad or whoever is responsible for these children.

Many times, we sabotage our kids in the name of love. We feed them much more then they need and more often than not, it's high calorie foods. We place a cookie jar on our counters full of delicious looking cookies for the taking. In today's society, many times it is just easier to stop at a drive-through than to cook. The problem is, it gets to easy and becomes an everyday thing. We obviously don't know what we are doing to them, or we would stop doing it.

It's hard to believe that today's society could be so uninformed. Many are setting their kids up for a lifetime of pain—physically, mentally, and emotionally. Like I said before, it takes work on our part to find the right food, cook it, and serve it in an appealing way.

Are you willing to give time to keeping your family healthy? Our kids are under our care for maybe eighteen years.

This is our opportunity to train them in the way they should go. We teach them to brush their teeth and keep clean. We teach them to not run into the street, eat worms, or drink and drive. Why? Because all of these can bring harm to them. Yet, we so easily give them money and send them to a greasy fast-food place to fill their bodies with unhealthy choices. Then, we pray for them not to get sick and to live a long life! *What's wrong with this picture?*

∽

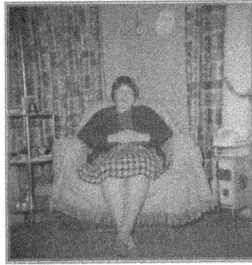

~ 9 ~

Two Hundred Pounds And Gaining

By the sixth grade, my weight had reached close to 200 pounds, according to the school nurse's loud announcement. That hit the playground like front-page news. Those were not good times. The kids ridiculed me for days. All I wanted was to be normal. Whatever that was.

I thought God must have really been mad at me to make me like this. What bad thing could I have done to deserve this life of abuse? It felt like it anyways. I'm sure at that age I didn't know what abuse was, but looking back, that is exactly what it was. I began to hate school with a passion, not participating in anything. As a result, I failed the sixth grade and having to take it over again made me the biggest kid once again. I'm not saying that all overweight children fail. I am telling you what happened to me. If it happened to me, it could happen to any overweight or obese child.

∾

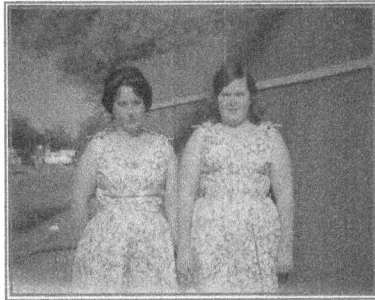

10

Shopping

Iremember going shopping for school clothes. *Oh my!* Mother screamed all day, and I cried non-stop. I barely was able to slip into a size twenty two-and-a-half dress. To make things worse, we had to go to the "old lady" section in the stores. You can imagine what I looked like.

My dear, sweet mother really helped things when she cut my hair so short that I looked like a boy. That went really well with all my big red freckles.

I think that was about the time that I asked God to either make me normal or kill me! And I was very serious. I didn't know God personally, but I knew He was out there somewhere, and He could put me out of my misery.

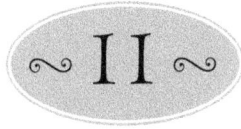

~ II ~

Stupid Diets

I tried every diet known to man. Can you imagine an eleven-year-old searching for the latest fad diet? My efforts led me to the rice diet, vegetable diet, juice diet, and don't forget the grapefruit diet. On all these diets you don't get anything but that particular food for a long time. They were deadly, but I didn't know it. I just heard that I could lose weight if I did them. Of course, nothing worked. I was so starved after the diets; it caused me to eat everything in sight. And you guessed it ... I gained even more weight.

The thought of killing myself became constant. Thank the Lord, even though I didn't know Him, He knew me, and He had a plan for my life. It was very difficult at that time imagining any kind of future for myself.

In my mind, there wasn't any way to stop this madness except for death. I needed help, but no one around me seemed to know what to do, and it was easier not to think about it. Somehow, it just wasn't a priority, and besides, I would grow out of it, right?

~

12

Making It Through Heartbreaking Years

Somehow, making it through junior high and losing a few pounds didn't make a difference in how I was treated.

In the seventh grade, when walking to class, a boy named Randy, ran up and hit me in the back. It knocked the breath out of me. He spat on me and said some very unkind things, then ran away. I hadn't done anything to cause him to dislike me so much. But it did make the other kids laugh so I suppose he accomplished his goal. Today this type of bullying would be considered a hate crime.

Some of the teachers had no mercy. They made wisecracks about me all the time. I remember once in a junior high Physical Education class, I fell on the blacktop and hit my head. My eye was bleeding, and the gym teacher asked me if *I had broken the blacktop!* Of course everyone laughed. What is the matter with people? It sure seemed people were heartless.

We really need to teach our kids to be kind to others, no matter what. Much of the time kids are cruel because that's what they learn at home. I do understand that hurting people, hurt people. Still, it's a parents job, if at all possible, to teach kindness as well as ABCs. And if your own child is overweight, don't call them names. You may think you can shame them into losing weight, but you can't. You will only do further harm to their self-image and self-esteem.

I can remember many days walking home crying because of something someone did or said just to hurt me and make others laugh. I was ashamed all of the time. I was given advice on a regular basis. The advice was always the same: "Just *lose the weight*—that's *all you gotta do.*" "Just *go on a diet.*"

When you see, or if you know, a "fat person," don't just assume that they eat all the time, and don't assume that they haven't tried to lose the weight. Don't be so quick to judge them. You probably don't know the facts. Things are not always as they seem. Sometimes we assume that an overweight person must set around and stuff their face all the time. Much of the time it's not the amount of food eaten, it's the type of food eaten. Some people become carb sensitive. The more carbohydrates like breads, pasta, sugar, white potatoes, and the likes, cause some people to gain weight. Our bodies will burn carbs before it will burn fat. Therefore the fat remains and is stored up for when the body runs out of carbs. If we keep eating a high amount of carbs, we never burn the unwanted fat. This is why very low carbs, high protein diets work well.

∽

~ 13 ~

Ashamed

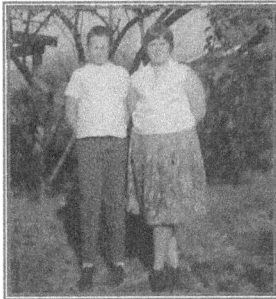

My own brothers were ashamed of me, and who could blame them? We all went to the same school. They were overweight at this time but not obese and didn't have a clue what I was going through.

We had to walk a mile or so to school and back, and most of the time I walked alone. It doesn't seem like much of a walk now, but as I said, the girls had to wear dresses to school and my legs were so big they rubbed together causing some serious chafing and constant pain.

I would sweat like crazy and my face turned red. That must have been a lovely sight. My own shame outweighed anything others thought about me, to be sure.

Again, I just didn't know what to do. I only knew how I felt. I certainly didn't need the help of others to make me feel unlovely and unaccepted. I could do that by myself.

~

~ 14 ~

Listen

I really hope people are listening to me and will have the guts to stop their children from becoming me.

Please take the steps that are needed to save your child from this incredible, unnecessary pain and embarrassment. I understand how sad my story seems, and it was, but don't lose sight of the reason it's being told. The more you know and understand the ramifications of obesity, the more you can do to help your child, or you yourself, avoid it. I'm here to tell you, it hurts.

There were many heartbreaking times for me in junior high and high school. We had to participate in Physical Education. Oh yeah ... that would be the end of me for sure!

It wasn't so much the fact that I couldn't do the running and jumping, or that I was always the last one picked for everything. It wasn't even the fact that the teachers made fun of me. What I really dreaded was "Shower Time," when I had to take my clothes off in front of all those skinny girls. It was devastating. Even my so-called friends would chime in with the name-callers. I ended up just taking an "F" in PE instead of taking the ridicule. It just seemed like the easiest way out.

Nowadays, schools don't even make the kids shower. They might smell bad, but certainly, less pain and ridicule are afflicted on the overweight kids because they are not exposed to the what the world would call, "normal-sized" kids.

~

15

No Date For The Fat Girl

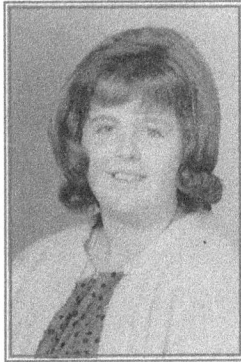

We must not forget the dances, parties, and ball games that I was never invited to. Does it sound to you like I had somewhat of a lousy childhood? Well, as a matter of fact, I did.

My hope is that this book will somehow open the eyes of those responsible for the precious overweight children and teens in this world. They could easily go through the same things I did, unless somebody helps them. And, in this day and age, kids don't just think about killing themselves—they do it. We should all be doing our best to make sure *over weight* never becomes a problem to start with.

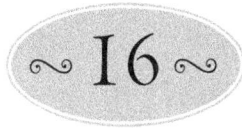

~ 16 ~

Fast-Food Fix

As I mentioned before, we teach our kids to take a bath, brush their teeth, and comb their hair; we warn them not to smoke or hang around with bad people. But many times, we forget to teach them that eating the wrong things could make their lives a living hell.

We give them money and send them off not having a clue what they're putting in their bodies. Sometimes we do know what they're eating, but don't have the time or the energy to address it. We might as well just tell the truth here. A lot of parents are just too busy.

Let us not be a part in weakening our children physically and emotionally. What kind of example have we been to our kids? We can always be a better example, right?

There is nothing more important than your family. Teach them to do the right things while they're young. Teach them to respect themselves enough to do the right things even when no one is watching them. Teach them to form the proper habits in everything they do. I believe most people know right from wrong and we very much need to pass that on to our children.

If we don't teach them to do what's right, someone else will teach them to do the wrong things. We can just about count on it. While our kids are in our home, it's our call. When they leave our home, it becomes their decision. What they learn now will continue with our grandchildren. Allow me to refer to the Bible, it tells us to,

"Train up a child in the way he should go: and when he is old, he will not depart from it" (Proverbs 22:6).

I know you love your children. We are all busy, and sometimes it's hard to find answers. It can be very hard to say *no*. We've learned to *'just say no,'* to drugs. Why not *'just say no,'* to unhealthy food? We, as parents, might need to be retrained ourselves in the area of eating before we can help the ones we love. It is very important that we be willing to learn and change.

We can save the generations to come by changing our thinking about what we eat and feed our families.

༄

~ 17 ~

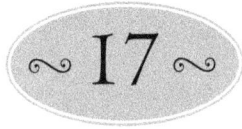

Don't Turn Me Off

Please, hear my heart. I'm not trying to be hard. I just know what I'm talking about. When I see overweight kids walking down the street, or if I'm watching TV programs about two-year olds who weigh 150 pounds, it hurts me greatly. The mothers say they don't know why little Johnny is so fat. The mother then unashamedly lists all that she has fed him in a day. What in the world is she thinking?

We can probably assume the mother never had the right training as a child. A lack of knowledge is one way obesity is passed on from generation to generation. It needs to stop. There needs to be more awareness and information about obesity and the connection with health problems in children. I think if more parents knew the facts about obesity's connection with diabetes, liver, lungs, and musculoskeletal complications, there might be more change in the homes where eating is concerned. As I stated before, in the past thirty years childhood obesity has tripled according to the, National Center for Chronic Disease Prevention and Health Promotion. **"We are seeing more concerns of Coronary Heart disease, as well as Thyroid and metabolism up-sets in very young children. Educate the parents, and the children will live more healthy."**

❦ 18 ❦

High School Dropout

When I was in the tenth grade, I lost a little weight, but again, it just didn't seem to make a difference. My grades were falling, and I cut school so much that my parents just allowed me to drop out altogether. They didn't understand my actions were because of the struggles with the obesity stigma. They couldn't know what I was enduring at school. They just knew my grades were falling and I was becoming hard-hearted and lifeless.

Parents, please see the signs. Talk to your kids and really listen to them. Ask them what they are feeling. Inquire about their day at school. Read between the lines. Don't settle for yes and no answers. Be creative and nosey. Are they spending more time alone? Check for hidden food in their room. Are you watching their weight? Maybe you should. Are you aware of what they should weigh? Get involved. I know it will take extra time and effort on your part. There is nothing more important in this life than your children. I can't tell you how many times I wanted to take my own life. God was watching over me. Someone must have been praying. Don't wait until it's too late. Do something now. Protect your treasures ... your kids!

❦

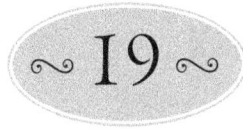

~ 19 ~

The Search

Now the real diet quest began. As I mentioned before, I tried many diets, which included the apple diets, fruit diets, the low-calorie diets, and anything else I found out about. I even tried the cigarette diet. I knew it was crazy, but I started smoking instead of eating. Believe it or not, I did lose some weight. It didn't matter that I could die of lung cancer as long as I lost the weight. What was I thinking?

When I was eighteen, I had my first date and I married him. I lost a bit more weight before the wedding so that I could fit into a size twelve wedding gown. The marriage didn't last. Neither did my weight loss. My divorce had nothing to do with my weight, he was just a jerk, plain and simple. The weight did come back because my eating habits had never changed.

I didn't understand that I needed to change the entire way I ate and the way I thought about food. Food is for nutrition, not a painkiller. Most people know food can become a comforter for mental pain. The problem is, if you don't find out how to get the root of the pain stopped, you keep using the food to ease the hurt. More food, more weight, more pain.

I gained and lost weight for years, and like everyone else, each time that I would gain the weight back, it would be more than the time before. I was at a total loss of what to do. Now I was a fat divorcee with a baby, and I smoked. Could it get much worse?

~ 20 ~

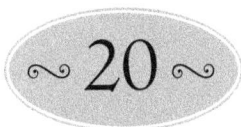

Lose The Weight Or Get Lost

Once again, I met a man that wanted to date me, but he couldn't handle the fat (you see, I did have a great personality, and I had a pretty face). His friends would tease him so much that he told me if I wanted to date him, I would need to lose the weight. I went on a starvation diet and began to lose weight quickly. Yet, it seemed that I could never lose enough to please people. I always needed to lose a bit more. I thought I was looking pretty good at 155. I'm 5'7 but according to my doctor I still needed to lose another thirty pounds or so. According to the boyfriend, I needed to drop a whole lot more. I would continue to search for answers to many things in life. I knew I could lose the weight now, but I didn't know how to keep it off yet.

∾

~ 21 ~

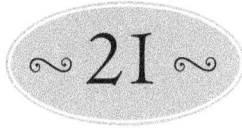

The Beginning Of New Life

In 1971, I met someone else. He totally changed my life. His name is Jesus Christ.

My life was about to be turned around so much that I wouldn't even recognize it. From one day to the next, things were different.

I received Jesus Christ as my Lord and Savior. I died to my old self and was born again. My thinking was somehow different. I had asked Jesus to come into my heart and change my life.

My boyfriend didn't receive my new lifestyle very well and asked me to choose between him and God. I didn't know God very well, but I knew that there was no contest here. God was my life now, with or without my friend. We didn't stay together long after that.

I began to learn about God and His Word, noticing a real change inside of me. My mind was being renewed. I found out quickly that although my spirit got saved, my body didn't. I gained all the weight back in a short time and didn't even realize it.

As a new Christian, not knowing very much about God, Jesus, or the Holy Spirit, I began to learn about the blessings that came with being saved. I found a church and was learning great things. I learned I could talk to God and He actually heard me. I learned that He wanted me to be alive and well, in every area of my life. I never knew how much God really did love me, fat and all. I found in

God's word that I could do all things through Christ who gave me strength. I could ask God for wisdom about everything.

Several years passed, and I got busy trying to support my daughter, Cindy, and going to school—just plain old life. I truly understand the challenges of being a single parent. Life can get hectic and sometimes we can easily get our priorities mixed up. I seemed to find less and less time for church which, for me, was a mistake. One learns so much after the fact. It is so important to strive for a firm foundation in any good thing we find for our lives. When wisdom comes, you can count on something always trying to steal it. Standing firm is a choice. I have made the wrong one too many times. Thank God we can do it again until we get it right.

❧

~22~

Life Goes On

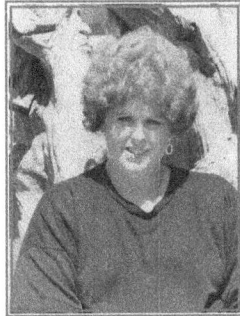

In 1978, I met Gerson, my second husband. We dated for a while, and I noticed that he never mentioned me being fat. He just kept telling me how beautiful I was. This was different! I thought, "I'd better hang on to this one."

We got married and lived happily ever after ... *Yeah right!* No, we have had our ups and downs, but we are still together after thirty-three years. Although, in the past, we have had many, many challenges because of my weight, our latter years have been much more peaceful. After being married even a couple of years, I kept thinking how strange it was that he never mentioned the fat. It was very nice for a change. It wasn't him with the fat problem, it was me.

In my quest to find the magic bullet that would make me thin, I became disgusted with all the many diets I tried. I thought, "Gerson loves me just the way I am, so why should I worry about it?"

As hard as I tried to be fat and happy, that nagging feeling would never leave me. My weight was always on my mind. It consumed me, right along with food. Food became my comforter more than ever.

Even though I wasn't going to church, I still prayed. God's love somehow helped me to know that He heard me when I prayed. I was very unhappy and disappointed with myself. I was embarrassed to go anywhere; I was a prisoner in an almost-300-pound body.

My thoughts would always turn towards the mental and physical pain that seemed never-ending. I didn't want go anywhere, do anything, or see anyone. I wouldn't look in a mirror because it reminded me of how big I had become. Cindy would be embarrassed of me if I needed to go to school to meet with her teachers. Shopping for clothes became a nightmare. I did enjoy food shopping. We never went out to eat because I just knew people would stare at me and wonder why I was eating, because surely I didn't need more food. It might have all been just something I perceived, but from past experience's, I knew how rude and unforgiving some people could be. This just couldn't go on. Something had to change, but just as before, I didn't know what to do. I felt myself becoming hard-hearted and cold once again. I couldn't see anything to live for. The devil will convince you that everyone would be better off without you.

Please do not lose sight of why I am telling you all of this. It's not for you to feel sorry for me. It's not so I can vent the past. It is a warning to those who might be headed for this kind of life. It's a wakeup call to parents and caregivers. The truth is; one person's pain can divert many from the same experience if heeded.

∾

23

Disgusted

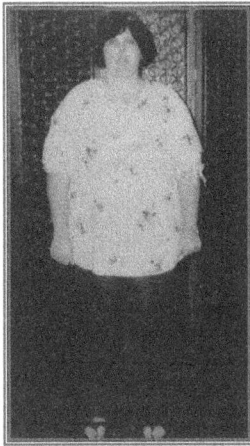

As I recall, it was the summer of 1981, in a small rental home in Norwalk, California, I was sitting in my big chair watching TV with a jar of peanut butter in one hand and a bag of chocolate chips in the other. (I was making my own peanut butter cups) I was hurt, disgusted, and food medicating. I didn't have a clue how to get out of the big mess parts of my life had become.

I was at my wits' end when I saw an advertisement on TV to join a woman's gym. At almost 300 pounds, exercise was not high on my list of fun things to do, but I took a chance and went to the gym. I got through the program that the skinny girl set up for me and headed for the spa!

God is so good. When I got to the spa, a woman named Carol was telling the other women in the spa how she had lost over 100 pounds. Well, my ears shot to attention! I wasn't shy about asking her to start at the beginning. I boldly asked her not to leave anything out.

Here's where it gets good. Carol told us how she and some of the women at her church were doing this new thing called *Free to Be Thin*, by Marie Chapian and Neva Cole. It was based on the Bible and prayer.

I asked my new friend Carol what kind of church they met at. When she told me where they met, I knew I couldn't go. You see, the church where I first attended after receiving Christ, warned me about *those* kinds of people—you know: the ones that rolled in the aisles and swung from the chandeliers, the charismatic people. At the time I didn't realize how judgmental that was. Hopeful that kind of teaching has changed.

Carol assured me that we would be meeting in the kitchen and no one would be swinging from anything.

I didn't really care what they did at this point, if they had the answer to my problem. I needed help, and these women were willing to do just that. I was desperate, and agreed to meet Carol that week for the meeting.

෯

~ 24 ~

They Knew My Pain

To my surprise, and in spite of my ignorance, the meeting was great. The women kept their feet on the ground and were all very nice. They seemed to know the pain I was in and seemed to have the answer.

I started the program the very next day. This was different from anything I had ever seen. The book said that I should pray and ask the Lord how much weight I needed to lose and what I should weigh.

According to the doctor's chart, I should have weighed in at about 125 pounds, tops. When a person is a whopping 290-something, 125 seems impossible. I did pray and believe that the Lord instructed me to concentrate on losing the first forty to fifty pounds. That I could see. I didn't hear God's voice, I just knew in my heart that was what I was supposed to do.

I began to cut my daily intake of calories down to 1,200. Everything that went into my mouth was counted. Those calories were spent like dollar bills. Believe me, I made every calorie count.

Was there still hunger? Oh yeah. Some days my body threw a fit, but I started to lose weight after the first week. That was so encouraging that I just kept it up.

As large as I was, I had to lose twenty to thirty pounds before people noticed anything, but I did, and they did begin to notice. It was exciting when people would ask, "Have you lost weight?" Talk about incentive. I stayed on that program for several months and lost about sixty-five pounds. At first, it was hard, but I got used to it quickly, and it became fun to spend my calories and get the most out of them. I was faithful with it and was becoming happy once again. I attended the weekly meetings and was weighed each week. Only one woman knew our weight. I liked that, even though there were very large women there just like me. If I remember correctly, it was a six to eight week program, long enough to get the hang of it and be able to do it on our own.

႙

❧ 25 ❧

Plateau

As time passed, I hit the plateau that we so often hear about, and I was stuck. At the time, everyone was talking about the medically supervised fasting diet. With this particular diet, you just drank a protein of some kind and didn't eat any solid food.

My friends, and my doctor suggested that I get on this new diet because of the plateau I had hit with the other diet programs. I did go on the fast, and in about three months, I became very ill. The doctors insisted that I must be eating something to be getting sick. There was no solid food allowed on this program. Also, with this prolonged fast, you couldn't eat certain things when you are coming off the fast. You could become very sick and could even die. I was not eating anything, but I was definitely sick.

There were many nights spent in the emergency room with horrible pain. Finally, they found the problem: it was my gall bladder. Immediate surgery was needed. The doctors that were overseeing the program wouldn't let me back on the fast, and that was okay with me! I did lose 50-60 pounds.

Still having much more weight to lose, I wondered where to go next. You see, when I stopped my fast, I gained a lot of the weight back. The wrong diet will do that to you every time. Wrong for me anyway. When you're not learning and preparing meals for yourself you don't seem to learn the changes that need to be made to maintain the weight loss. We'll learn more about this in a future chapter.

Many obese people lose their gall bladders. It is generally overworked with the large amount of food it must filter. If you don't have a gall bladder you really need to be very cautious. I needed to eat more live foods as well as more green leafy vegetables. I was told to avoid high fat foods and eat more whole grains and legumes. My pancreas is now my biggest filter. It is doing the work of the missing gall bladder as well as its own work.

So now, it was back to the drawing board for me. I needed to find a new plan, but I had developed a *never to give up* attitude.

༄

~ 26 ~

Getting To Know You!

One thing was for sure: I was getting to know my Heavenly Father better and better as the days went by. Remember the little church that hosted the diet club? Well, I decided to go to the church and see just what all the fuss was about.

Yep, I walked right in, sat down, and watched every move that went on. The people were weird, all right: they would come up and hug you and shake your hand. They all seemed happy. They sang songs that made me happy to be there. They seemed to really be in love with God and was very open with showing it. The songs they sang seem to be scriptures out of the Bible and touched me deeply. They had guitars, drums and other musical instruments. The other church had a piano and organ. This was all I had known. It was good, but there was just a different atmosphere in this new place of worship that drew me in. Even with all the peace in the place, I was never far from the nagging feeling of being obese.

My husband was not born again at that time, and he wouldn't even listen to "God stuff." He was a very hard person and anti-social. That caused a lot of fighting in our home. After about a year, I began to think about a divorce. The mental pain was too much to bear and I found myself using food as a comforter once again. Of course we all know what happened then. I gained weight. Although knowing God did not condone divorce, I couldn't keep on living like that. My daughter, Cindy, who was reaching her teen years was becoming nervous and upset a lot, with all the fighting. Enough was enough; divorce seemed to be the answer.

That Sunday morning, as I was in church, in the middle of the singing, my husband walked past me and sat in the front row of the church. I wasn't even aware that he knew where the church was. About halfway through the service, my husband got up, went to the altar, and fell on his knees and got radically saved. He willingly voiced his desire to let God change his life. There were tears and shouts of joy everywhere, even though no one knew him. Several of the men in the church went up, kneeled around him, and prayed with him. They truly showed great love for him.

Many times, it seems as if God waits until the very last second to show Himself. I just stood there in shock and probably a little disbelief.

೪

～ 27 ～

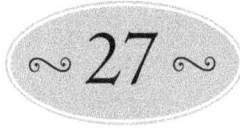

Wonderful Lord

What a wonderful God and Father we have. My husband and I stayed in that church for a few years.

We began to have a relationship with the Lord that we never knew existed. God has become very real to us ever since that day. Before, we knew of Him as God, now we were seeing Him, as not only God, but Father God. We began to read the Bible and found out about all the good things God had made available for us.

Things changed drastically. With God's help, we began to look at life differently. It always works better when a husband and wife are in agreement with one another. Now we were on the same side, God's side. Prayers were being answered, and life just got better and we seemed to breathe easier. I believe God was honoring the choices we were making together as Christians.

We had disagreements, but we were able to work them out. We knew that God was helping us, and we began to learn how to do things God's way. It was just better, easier, and without so much of the stress we'd had before.

Time and circumstances would move us to Cottonwood Christian Center in Los Alamitos, CA. It was quite a bit larger than the previous church. We became involved in the different ministries and began to serve as needed. My once very shy husband became an usher at nearly ever service. I served as department leader over the telephone ministry. We both graduated from the Cottonwood School of Ministry and continued to serve as needed. God was stretching us and it felt good. God has a way to set us up for success in all areas of life that concerns us. I have since become an ordained minister and have served as Administrator and Associate Pastor for a season, and have written mini books that have been distributed in many parts of the world. Our choice to serve God has changed our lives more than words can say.

Now back to the seemingly never-ending search for a way to lose weight and keep it off. Over the years, I have gained and lost hundreds of pounds. I still needed to find the key to unlock my answer. You might be wondering why God didn't just make it known so many years ago. I don't know. I'm sure He had a reason. Maybe He did and I just wasn't listening.

∾

∾ 28 ∾

Still Searching

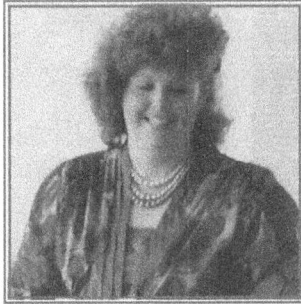

Still needing to lose quite a bit of weight, I learned about a weight-management program that was teaching people to change their life style. It was a diet program, but not just a diet. It was designed to teach people what to eat and when to eat. They taught me portion sizes along with good low-fat and low-calorie recipes. The one question the diet counselors asked was, "Why do you eat?"

In thinking about it, I realized that I ate all the time and not just because of hunger. I ate when I was happy, when I was sad, and when I was in emotional pain. I ate when I got mad at my husband, and I ate when we made up. There was never a lack of a reason to eat. Food was an obsession to me and had been as far back as I could remember.

On every diet, my focus was always on the food. A doctor once said, "If you ask a thin person how often they think about food, most of the time the answer would be, they only think about food when they're hungry." So what happened to me?

My brothers, John and Dennis, and I had been programmed as children to eat, eat, eat. Now I needed to somehow undo all the wrong teaching and start over. This program suggested I attended weekly meetings for support. I never missed and was diligent about everything they asked me to do. They asked me to keep a diary of every bite consumed, how much, and what time it was eaten, and how I felt at that time. I exercised regularly and never cheated. *Never!* This was serious for me.

By the way, my parents and both brothers had also become very obese. We children were trained the same way, and the bad habits caught up with them as well. Since my mom and dad were eating the same as we did, they developed incorrect eating habits, as well, which led to obesity.

Growing up, we were forced to clean our plates. We were told that children were starving in China, so we needed to eat everything. Sometimes I wondered just how many kids in China I single-handedly saved from starving to death by cleaning my plate. The problem was that I learned to *enjoy* cleaning my plate—and everyone else's.

༄

29

Bad Habits Are Easy To Learn ... Hard To Break

I'm sure you've heard it all before, but you haven't heard it from me. Maybe my story will be the one that sets something off in you and brings about change. Maybe it will encourage you to pay closer attention to what you feed your children.

It's strange how most people never think of food becoming an addiction. A person can become addicted to different foods as well as drugs and alcohol. I've always wondered, though, why we never get addicted to spinach, broccoli, or tofu! Hmmm! No, the things I became addicted to are sweets, breads, and trans-fats. As a child, these are the very things I was taught to, and even forced to, become addicted to by eating too much of them.

There were so many things to learn about nutrition, portion size, and how to retrain my taste buds to like the *good for you foods*. It's never too late; you can start today, even if it's Tuesday. Monday never comes when you're starting a diet!

The Bible tells us that God's people are destroyed for lack of knowledge. My parents were no exception. Lack of knowledge can become a death trap. The crazy thing is that once you're addicted to wrong things, you can receive all the knowledge on the planet and not be able to change without proper help and support. Knowledge without the wisdom to use it, and action to make it happen, is useless.

~ 30 ~

Parent/Guardian Responsibility

Please understand that I am not a doctor, dietitian, or psychiatrist. I am one who has lost over 150 pounds without surgery and kept most of it off for over 20 years. I still deal with a few extra pounds now and then and will always be cautious of what, and how much, I eat.

Remember those fat cells that never go away? They cry out to be fed, but we cannot give in to our flesh. It is a dangerous thing to do in any area of our lives.

Do I want to eat everything in sight occasionally? Oh yeah. But do I? No. This would only cause more pain and stress. Most of the time I eat *what* I want, but never *all* I want. Moderation and wisdom is key.

Think about it: it's your mind that wants more, not your body. I've noticed that my grandson will eat plenty and be asking for more. We insist that he wait for a while before having anything else, and most of the time, he forgets about it. Give your brain time to catch up with your stomach. You'll find that after you get your mind off food, you are quite satisfied with what you've had. I believe the only way we can keep our flesh under submission is to trust and depend on God. This is our responsibility.

I was obese as a child, and according to the doctors, was still considered obese and overweight most of my life. My childhood was heartbreaking and unnecessary. I'll have to say, in all honesty and much love, that my parents were responsible for those years.

They were naïve and uninformed—but you and I are not. If you, as parents, see signs of obesity in your child, get help. Do all that you can do to find the problem and the answer. Don't dismiss seventy-five pounds at age five as baby fat. Do the responsible and loving thing, and *get your child help now. Ask your doctor for help. Don't take no for an answer. Check out obesity web sites, talk with friends.* The fact that you have this book is encouraging. My email address is available to you as well. lois@youcantakeyourlifeback.org

Always remember, the problem could very well be a medical one. You won't know unless you check it out. Many things could be a factor in this.

The thyroid gland, as well as the hypothalamus gland, could need some adjusting. Again, I am not a doctor, but I have studied the hypothalamus gland. It has a big part in the body's heat, sleep, and hunger regulation among others. It has been said that if this gland is not working properly, a person can be hungry all the time, even right after eating a good-sized meal. This was true for me. After eating a meal, I would be starving within a half an hour. The hunger pangs were so severe that I would have to eat something else. I know many people that have experienced the same feelings.

Many doctors overlook the connection between the continual hunger and the hypothalamus gland. This information could be critical for you to know. More information will be given in a later chapter.

◠◡

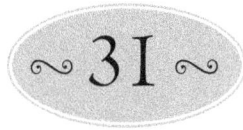

～ 31 ～

Faithful

Well, I stayed on this new eating program for about a year and was faithful to all that the counselors said needed to be done. I walked with my friend Linda almost every day during that year. She was into walking, bike riding, and rock climbing, and she kept me going.

At the end of that year, my weight loss was 110 pounds, and I wore a size ten dress. My weight was 149 pounds—for about ten minutes!

Family and friends were beginning to tell me that I looked sick, and the doctors still said I was overweight according to their charts. I can't tell you how depressing it was to hear that after all the hard work I had done.

My pride was quickly squashed by well-meaning people. It just wasn't enough. Would it ever be enough? And could I keep the weight off? You see, going back to eating my own cooking, the weight started to come back on.

For one year, I had eaten prepackaged foods that contained the right portions and calorie amounts. The cost of these types of programs are quite expensive and I no longer could stay on it. Now I was on my own again, and thinking on my own. I gained about fifteen pounds and leveled off, and that was okay. I looked and felt good, but it was still very hard to keep my weight down. Most of my life has been an up-down challenge where weight was concerned. "When God, when, how God, how" were the questions.

∽

～ 32 ～

Thank You Lord

A s I said before, we had joined a new church and were getting
to know God, who He was, and why He loved us so much.
We learned about God's mercy and grace and how it had been
surrounding us in the many painful years of the past. He had been
there when I was teased by the other kids. His mercy had abounded
in all the times I prayed to die.

I'm glad now, of course, that God didn't grant me my prayer.
It makes me shudder to think of my destiny if I had died without
accepting Jesus as my Savior. God was good to me, even when I
didn't know it. How wonderful is that? His ways are definitely not
our ways. The Bible tells us in Romans 5:8, "While we were still
sinners, Christ died for us." Why is it that we take so long to know
God as He is? He is *love*—the Bible tells us so. As a child I thought
I must have done something to make Him mad at me. It's sad that
it took me so many years to find out about His unconditional love.

The more I became acquainted with God the Father and His
Words to me, the less I began to dwell on my weight, my looks,
and what others thought of me. My main focus had turned to
something that would fill my hunger better than food.

The Spirit of God and the goodness of knowing Him had
somehow changed me. You see, when we receive God's Son, Jesus
Christ, as our Savior, we are adopted into God's household,
(Galatians 4:4-7). We become heirs according to the promise that
God made to Abraham in Galatians 3:26-29. Again, a lack of
knowledge can stop us from reaching our goals in life. We can be

as born again as the next guy, but if we are ignorant of what Bible says, we won't know what we're missing out on.

When a person is adopted into an earthly family, they become an heir to the head of that household. In other words, they are in the *will.* It's the same with being adopted into God's family. We are heirs of Christ. We are in the *will.* Do you know what the *Will* says? We need to find out just what comes in the adoption packet. We can easily find out. Jesus left us a copy of His Last Will and Testament when He died. It's called … the Bible.

Don't be intimidated by the Bible. Once you ask Jesus into your heart, the Holy Spirit becomes your guide. I hear many people say they tried to read the Bible but just couldn't understand it. If you are not born again, you won't understand it. How can a person understand the things of God if he doesn't belong to God? Once you have Christ and the Holy Spirit living within you, you become enlightened in the things of God. The power of God dwells in you and causes you to comprehend things that you wouldn't have comprehended before receiving Christ.

The Bible is our instruction book for life, and we will find answers for everything that we will ever go through in this life. The question is, *Will you take the time to find the answers?* Is it worth it to search until you finally do? How dedicated and driven are you to find out what God, our Creator, has instructed you to do? The search might take a lifetime, and you will never find all the answers this side of heaven.

෨

33

You're In The Will

My parents died several years ago and left a will. Now, if I had never read that will, I would have never known that they left me everything, much to my surprise. Don't miss the point here.

Everyone needs to read the Will that God has left us. It's the greatest thing you will ever read. When you do read it, every time you come across the word "whosoever," replace it with your name. You are the "whosoever" the Bible is referring to. Just like in a natural will, you will benefit from the death of the departed. That's just how it is. Unless a seed dies, and is planted in the ground, fruit will not grow from the seed.

Jesus had to die in order for us to receive what He left for us in the Will. His resurrection from the dead was the beginning of new life for all that believe in Him. And we will receive what He has purchased for us: everlasting life with Him.

Many people have never read the Will. They don't have a clue what belongs to them. They suffer through life being sick, broke, sad, and lonely, all because they don't know what belongs to them. I was one who just didn't know. I was twenty years old before anyone ever told me about Jesus. Once I heard the truth, I received Him as my Lord and Savior immediately. I had no reason to wait any longer.

I needed my life to change big time. I had no direction. I was spinning like a top, out of control. I had a child, no job, and was on welfare. I got a Bible right away and started reading. That was in

1971, and I've been reading it ever since. Many times I had to read repeatedly for it to sink in, but it finally did. It really is like a light bulb coming on. Believe it or not, I never get tired of reading the Bible. I learn something new every day.

෧ර

∾ 34 ∾

God Had A Plan

What does this have to do with fat, food, and weight? There is only one way to achieve the things in life that God has promised to us. We need to revere God and find out what His will is for us. God will let us live out our lives in His permissive will, but all the time desiring for us to benefit from being in His *perfect* will. He holds nothing back from us. It is God's will for us to be in perfect peace. It's His will for us to live our lives with a healthy body and a sound mind. He wants us well and whole and He wants us to have nothing missing and nothing broken.

The Bible says in III John 1:2 "Beloved, I pray that you may prosper in *all things* and be in health, just as your soul prospers."

We all know that to be in good health, one thing we need to do is eat the right things. And it's pretty much a given that a continual diet of soda and candy bars are not going to produce good health. We know that a diet of fast food, cake, and ice cream is what got us in the place we're in now. Just like everything in this world, we have choices to make, and with choices come consequences, good or bad.

When I was a child, my choices were limited due to age and knowledge. It seems to me now, I was up against a stacked deck, and I was reaping for someone else's bad choices. Being fat as a child wasn't my fault, but becoming aware of what was happening gave me more ability to make better choices for myself. It just took a while before I figured it out. I hope this book will shorten that time for you.

As an adult, I had the power to change things. With God's help, I did just that, and you can too. Save yourself and your children from the mental and physical destruction that a life of obesity can hold.

There isn't one thing in this book about food that you probably don't already know. We all know that the food God intended for us to eat, is the food that He knew would be good for us. He made us, and He knows what it takes to keep us well and full of energy. He knew what foods would stop all the diseases that would soon come upon this earth. Man just got too smart for his own good. We figured out how to make all kinds of unhealthy things out of what God meant for our good. God gave us flour for bread, not cake and cookies. He gave us chicken, and we made deep-fried chicken strips. He gave us milk; we made shakes. He gave us potatoes, and we made chips. *I think you get my point.* Man has managed to pervert the goodness of the Lord in many ways, including our food.

෬

∾ 35 ∾

God's Perfect Will

There are many people hurting physically and emotionally because of being overweight or obese. I don't believe it's God's will for anyone to live with physical or emotional pain, although we sometimes do, it's not God's will. According to John 10:10, The thief (satan) comes to steal, kill, and destroy. But Jesus came that we may have abundant life. I'm sure everyone has their opinion and this is mine. I know that I wouldn't want my kids to live in any kind of pain. I don't believe God does either. It's a fact that the more overweight someone is, the more they are susceptible to diabetes, joint problems, and coronary issues. This is *not* God's perfect will for anybody's life.

I have had people weighing over 300 pounds tell me that they feel great and can do anything they want. I'm not sure they're telling the entire truth. They complain that their knees and backs hurt, and they can't walk out to the car for the third bag of groceries without having to rest between trips. They can't play with their kids, and it's hard to get in and out of the car, let alone go on a long trip. They have high blood pressure and probably an over-worked gall bladder. Yeah, this is feeling great.

I'm not saying that all overweight people have all of these problems, but most of them have some of these health issues. If we knew how much harder our heart has to pump for every pound we are over our ideal weight, we wouldn't believe it.

Just what is your ideal weight? You need to be realistic. If you're a 5' 2" woman, you know 170 pounds is too much. Now a woman 5' 10" could be okay at that weight.

If you belong to God, and you really want to know what's right for you, just ask, be silent, and listen. God will talk to you on the inside. You'll hear Him, and God is the best judge—not your skinny neighbor, your doctor, spouse, or your kids. You can't even trust yourself, and you know it!

Let me also say that not everyone was created to be what the world calls *thin* or *normal.* There is no such thing as normal, just opinions. There are a great number of thin people that eat terribly. They just have a metabolism that is much faster than others. They are still susceptible to the same diseases as everyone else.

Sometimes you will hear a thin person boasting about how much they can eat and not gain weight. No matter who's doing it, gluttony is a sin according to God. A thin person is in error if they are not willing to do the right things. They can be just as unhealthy as an overweight person and sometimes even unhealthier. Their bad moves are just not as noticeable as others.

Here is a word of caution: after you lose your weight, never get the idea that you can now eat all you desire. This is a lie straight from hell. You cannot, I repeat, *cannot* ever think you can go back to the old eating habits and remain at your proper weight. It might not show right away, but beware, it will show up, and you will be the first to know it. All of the sudden, your pants won't fit! It's a bad feeling!

❧

∾ 36 ∾

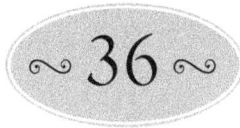

Are You Willing?

So, what's it going to take to get to the place where you are at your best? *A lot.* In my case, it took a lot of trusting in God to direct me, and a lot of time listening and obeying what I heard Him say inside my spirit. It took a lot of self-discipline and a lot of telling my flesh: *"No,* you can't have that" or *"No,* you can't have *all* of it, but you can have a piece of it." You see, your flesh is like a little child that wants its own way all the time. That child has to be trained to do the right thing.

We all need to have discipline or we will get into trouble or get hurt. In most cases with people being overweight, it's a matter of needing to be retrained. Personally, I had to get rid of so much wrong teaching and bad habits that it took me a long time. It was hard to rethink my whole life.

One very important thing is to never, ever give up. If you do, you may die young and unfulfilled. That would be a great loss. I know right now, if you're overweight and miserable, you're probably thinking that it might not be such a big loss if you weren't here. *Stop it right now!* You are dear to your family, friends, and to God. Things will change! You'll see. You do have much to give this world, and you will. Besides that, I'll bet you have a pretty face. Wow, how many times did I get told that? But you know what? I did! And so do you. God made us and He is proud of His creation. Things can only get better if you don't give up.

Be willing to listen and search for the answers you need for you or your child. Be willing to make changes where they need to be made. Getting informed takes time and energy but I can tell you, it's worth it.

❧

~ 37 ~

In Retraining

As a child, I was trained to eat everything on my plate, or I would get no dessert. It didn't matter that I was full—I needed to eat everything. You might want to think twice about insisting that your child cleans his/her plate and try not to make dessert a bribe.

What was happening to me? My stomach was being trained to hold more and more unnecessary food. The more food I took in, the more I desired. You probably know exactly the feeling I'm describing. It was like getting pregnant with fat cells, and remember, the thing about fat cells is that they know how to multiply and divide, but they've never learned to subtract! Even when you lose weight, you don't lose the fat cells. They just shrink and wait to be overfed once again. It may not seem very fair, but it's the truth—according to man's way of thinking, anyway.

Did you know that God thinks differently than we do? He can change things with just one word. The Bible tells us in Isaiah 55:8-9, "For My thoughts are not your thoughts, Nor are your ways My ways," says the Lord. "For as the heavens are higher than the earth, So are My ways higher that your ways, And My thoughts than your thoughts." God's word can change our thinking, our thinking can change our speaking, and our speaking can change our life. Mark 11:23-24 says, "For assuredly, I say to you, whoever says to this mountain, 'Be removed and be cast into the sea,' and does not doubt in his heart, but believes that those things he says will be done, he will have whatever he says. "Therefore I say to you, whatever things you ask when you pray, believe that you receive them, and you will have them." I have found over the years that the best place to be is on God's side. It works so much better than my way of doing things.

One important thing to remember is not to be stubborn. God is right every time, so don't argue about things. Just do things *His* way, and win. I know there will be some people that read this and think I am nuts. Oh well, staying on God's side is working for me just fine. It's always your choice.

∾

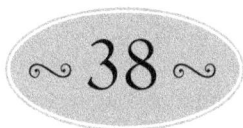

~ 38 ~

But God

Aᴄᴄᴏʀᴅɪɴɢ to God, I can call those things that do not exist, as though they do. In Romans 4:17 God does this very thing, and in Ephesians 5:1, the Bible tells us to be imitators of God. What exactly does that mean? It means that if you belong to God, you have the right to claim what the Bible says. God tells us to speak to those things that do not exist and call them into existence. If this is true, and it is, we have the right to call our fat cells to be the way God created them to be. We don't have to receive what man's facts tell us. We need to receive what the truth of God's Word tells us. You see, facts are always subject to change, but the truth of God can never change.

Remember, Mark 11:23-25 talks about speaking and believing in your heart. Do you see how important saying or speaking God's word really is? If God gave us permission to do what He does and say what He says, we should be doing it the best we can.

Now, please don't get me wrong here. I'm not saying that you can, "name it and claim it," or "blab it, and grab it." That is not what Mark 11:22–24 says. You can't just say it with your mouth—you must believe it in your heart, not your head, and it needs to be God's Word. This will take some practice, but if you will begin to speak God's Word over yourself, out loud so that you can hear it, it will eventually drop into your heart, and you will believe it. What you have already prayed will become a reality.

In order to have the promises of God work for us, we must follow the instructions that God has set up for us in His Word. I can teach a parrot to say, "I am a dog," but it will never become a dog because it will never believe that it is a dog. You have to do more than say what you want. Your heart has to believe what your mouth is saying. This could also work for the negative things you say as well, if you believe it in your heart. What you have been saying and believing, is most likely what you are having right now. Think about it.

The Bible tells us, "So then faith comes by hearing, and hearing by the Word of God" (Romans 10:17). You can say it like this: Faith comes when you continually hear the Word of God. No matter how you say it, faith comes. In fact, faith will also come if you are listening to yourself speak negative things. You will build up faith in those negative words and receive the consequences of it. So, if you get up every day and tell yourself, "I'm fat and ugly, and I will never make it in life," you could eventually be just that: a fat, ugly, nobody. And that's not how God intended you to live your life.

God tells us that in Christ, we are more than conquerors. He tells us that we can do all things through Christ who strengthens us. With God on our side and His Words in our mouth, we will win the battle with obesity.

Remember, this is not a game, and it's not easy. It takes practice and persistence. Also, it will take you believing in yourself plus, I have found that depending on the Lord greatly helps. There will be times of discouragement, and you might even want to quit. *Don't!* These feelings will pass. Talk to yourself, and tell yourself that you are doing great, God is on your side, you are a winner, and you will succeed! Take a deep breath, and keep doing the right things.

❧

～ 39 ～

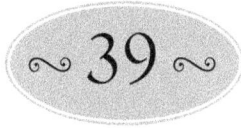

Be Like Your Father

We talked about Ephesians 5:1 and how to be imitators of God. Some might remember the song by Amy Grant, called "My Father's Eyes." It talks about looking at things through God's eyes. We need to see ourselves as the Lord sees us.

What do you see when you look in the mirror? Chances are, you don't see what God sees. I am fifty-nine years old and I have caught myself saying things like, "I feel like I am twenty until I look in the mirror." I needed to get my heart and mouth to line up. My heart was saying, "I feel so good, and I have so much energy," but my mouth was saying, "You're old and sad looking." I quickly changed my evil ways and words.

Did you know that God calls negative speaking *evil?* He does.

～

~ 40 ~

The Spies

Take a look in your Bible at Numbers 14:37. This is a true story about twelve spies that God sent into the land of Canaan to check out the situation. God had already told the Israelites that He had given them this land flowing with milk and honey. The problem was that most of them did not believe His promise.

Numbers 13 tells us these twelve men went out to see just what it would take to possess the land. You see, most of the time when God gives us a promise, He will also give us instructions as well. He told the Israelites *go and possess the land. I will give it to you if you will take it.* In other words, He told them, "I will, *if* you will." Anyhow, the twelve guys went to spy on the land that God had already said they could have. When they came back, ten of the men said, there was no way they could take the land. They said these guys were so big and bad that they thought they look like grasshoppers in their sight. This was not what God said, and was not a good confession (report). On the other hand, two of the spies, Joshua and Caleb, gave a different report. Their report was that they were well able to take the land. They knew that it didn't matter *how big* the other guys were! *God* had said that they could take the land, and they put their faith in *His Word*, not in what they saw with their eyes. The point is, we need to agree with God, even if the majority says something else. Our confession, or what we say, should never be contrary to what God says.

Another point is, God called the ten spies' report evil because it didn't line up or agree with His Word. So, if we want God on our side, we need to agree with Him. It is our job to find out what His

Word says and agree with it. First of all, God says in John 15:7: "If you abide in Me, and My words abide in you, you will ask what you desire, and it shall be done for you."

What is He saying here? He's asking us to take the time to read His book, talk to Him, and get to know Him, and then we will know what He wants for us.

If we are faithful in doing what God asks us to do, He will see to it that we get the answer that we desire. Understand God is not playing with us. He wants us to prosper even more than we do ourselves. The one thing we need to be clear on, is that we have to abide by the guidelines and standards that He Himself has placed in the Bible. He can't break His Word or it would be sin. If He tells us something needs to be done in a certain way, then that is how we need to do it.

Stop trying to take short cuts. They will just get you lost. God will never instruct you wrong. He will help you to get the correct information. He will give you wisdom on how to appropriate it to get the best results in your weight loss or that of a family member.

If we can learn to do life the way the Creator designed us to, we will save ourselves a lot of heartache and pain. It just doesn't make any sense that a created thing thinks it is wiser than the Creator who made it. Does it? I wish I had learned this a lot sooner than I did. You can learn from my mistakes and have quicker success.

Whether you want to lose weight, be healed of a sickness or have all your needs met financially, God is your source. Nothing else will do. If we can depend on Him to meet all of our needs, stress would end. Again, I am not saying this will all be easy. In fact, it won't be easy. I'll tell you right now that it will most likely be hard. Maybe it needs to be said here that you can lose weight without God. You can live life without God, and that's always your choice. I will tell you, He certainly has made my life better and easier. My desire is to make God a part of all that I do in this life. If I can show you a better way to lose weight, or help you to help your kids lose weight with the help of God, I must do it. The choice is yours whether or not you accept my suggestions.

Knowledge, with wisdom, is a key in losing weight and keeping it off. A lack of knowledge will kill and destroy us, but where there is the right knowledge and wisdom, we can succeed at everything we set our hands to do. In the next section, we'll look at some of God's promises and how they can affect our lives.

৵

~ 41 ~

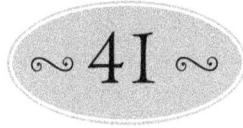

Promises Of God

PROMISE I

Philippians 4:13 "I can do all things through Christ who strengthens me."

We will need the strength of the Lord to stay on the right path. This is true in any area of our lives. We can try to lose weight on our own. Anyone can lose weight—just *don't eat!*

Of course, your hair will fall out, and your teeth might rot. Your kidneys will become weak, and in fact, every organ in your body may become sick and out of balance. You will lose weight, but you might even die.

Being successful, peaceful, and healthy in anything we do requires strength and wisdom from God. He tells us we *can* do all things through Christ, and the strength that comes into us when we receive Christ.

Obesity is twofold: it is a disease, but it can also be a sin. The sin part is gluttony. Gluttony is defined in part as over-indulgence of food or drink. We are hurting or defiling our body. Continued sin has consequences. In the case of continual overeating, the consequences could be heart, liver, or lung problems. Obesity could become a consequence which could led to diabetes, high blood pressure, and high cholesterol. Any one of these could lead to death.

In my case, and perhaps in your case, it was the upbringing and wrong training as a child that started the ball rolling. When we get old enough to know better, yet choose to continue with these uncontrolled habits, it becomes sin to us. I will refer to the Bible once again, which tells us, that to him who knows to do good and does not do it, to him it is sin (James 4:17). I think we all could be guilty of this, but we should strive to do the right things as soon as we realize our errors.

It's a sad thing to admit, but it's the truth. No matter how we would like to ignore it or pretend that it's not sin, it is. The one good thing is, we can be forgiven and start new. Thank God, He is a God of second chances. In fact, He will give us all the chances necessary for us to learn that He has the right answers.

I truly believe that in my quest to find out how to lose the weight and keep it off, I have found answers to many of my life's problems. Sometimes we learn things the hard way, but God can even use that to help us with our future. Still, I wish my parents had taught me differently. I really could have done without all the suffering.

Parents, I encourage you: don't let your children suffer the stigma of being obese. No matter how happy they seem to act, inside they are most likely hurting and scared. Help them to be healthy and to live long, strong lives. Show them that God is their answer and help in time of trouble. If we, as parents, have knowledge and wisdom, we can escape a lot of this life's pitfalls and expose them to our children as well.

One of a parent's jobs is to protect his or her children from harm. Sometimes we don't think about the abuse they may be taking from others outside the home. Many times, the abuse could go unseen, so we, as parents, need to pay attention to what our kids are saying, or not saying. As for me, I did tell my mom about the name calling and the hitting at school. I told her about being left out of things because of being fat. No action was taken. I finally just kept quiet. I stayed to myself. I only came out of my room when it was necessary. I begin to rebel about everything. I started to smoke, and hang around with a few bad kids that had other issues. Parents need to be nosey and insist on conversation. When things go this far, the only thing a parent can really do, is to get them help to lose weight. It's never too late to start. Yes, they may get mad at us now, but when they are older, they will honor and love us for watching after them and doing the right thing. We have to learn so we can teach.

PROMISE 2

I Corinthians 2:16(b) "But we have the mind of Christ."

Having the mind of Christ is, to most people, unthinkable. Most people can't comprehend that we have the power within us to make the right decision every time, in every situation. If God says we have the mind of Christ, then we do. If we choose not to exercise that right, God will not challenge our decision. We are free agents. But if we choose, we can have everything we need to live a healthy, successful life.

We have the manufacturer's handbook at our disposal, twenty-four hours a day (Bible). The biggest problem is that we don't open it. It just amazes me in my own life how many problems could have been solved a lot faster if I would have just gone to the Guidebook and read the instructions. God is so good, He gives us open-Book tests, and still, we refuse to turn the pages.

We all need to get busy.

PROMISE 3

James 4:2–3 "We have not, because we ask not, and when we do ask, we ask wrong."

So many times, we wait until the situation turns ugly, and only then do we beg God to fix it for us. Does this method work for you? It doesn't work for me.

Let's find out what God has promised, and then we can go to the throne room, present our petitions to the Lord, and walk away with thanksgiving and answers.

We can have great confidence in doing this. I John 5:14 says, "Now this is the confidence that we have in Him, that if we ask anything according to His will, He hears us. 15. And if we know that He hears us, whatever we ask, we know that we have the petitions that we have asked of Him." We do have the mind of Christ. We need to act on it.

PROMISE 4

II Corinthians 5:21 "We are the righteousness of God."

Assuming that you are born again, you are the righteousness of God. Receiving Christ restores us back to Father God. Adam's sin in the garden took that away. (If you are not born again, I encourage you to receive Christ right now. It will be the best thing you could do for yourself.) Just ask Jesus to forgive you of sin, come into your life and save you. Receive His sacrifice of death for you on the cross. Believe in your heart that God raised Him from the dead, and you will be saved (Romans 10:9-10).

To have the mind of Christ and the righteousness of Christ, you must have Christ. Life can be hard even with God on your side. I can't even imagine my life without God on my side. That is a horrifying thought.

This world is crazy, and we need the love and protection of the Almighty God. We need the great Salvation that Christ brings, and the comfort that the Holy Spirit brings to us the minute we say *yes* to Jesus.

When we receive Jesus Christ as our Lord and Savior, we receive right standing with God. Because Christ is righteous and comes to live in us, we become righteous because of Him. We can't earn it or be good enough for it. It is a free gift from God to the guilty, purchased with the Blood of Christ.

When you receive Christ and His righteousness, you receive full acquittal from all the charges of sin and iniquity against you. When you stand before the Mighty Judge on judgment day, you will be found "Not Guilty," all because you received Christ and His work on the cross.

Who in their right mind would turn that down? The righteousness of Christ gives you the right to petition God for the answer to obesity and anything else you need an answer for.

I don't know about you, but I have a lot of needs in my life other than losing weight. Good health, protection, provision, and forgiveness are great needs for us all. We need to succeed in all that we put our hands to do. My children need to succeed and be in great health. They need to be protected from harm and have wisdom and understanding of how to live life the best way they can.

We need to know how to please God. You and I losing weight is a small issue for God to deal with. He has all of the answers to all of life's situations. His answers are always right and free for the asking. Believe it or not, God is waiting for us to come to Him and receive what we need and want.

Many times we misjudge God as being a big, grouchy, mean God scanning the earth to find people who have messed up so that He can punish them. This idea is so far away from the truth!

You have probably heard the phrase, "God is love." Well, He *is* love, He *has* love, and He *gives* love. He is looking back and forth on the earth, but He's looking for someone to bless, not curse! He's looking for someone overweight to show His kindness to. The only thing He asks of us is that we come to Him. That's all … just come to Him. People are either too busy, too proud, or too "whatever" to just come. Is that you? Is that why nothing is happening in your life? When you're done doing it your way, give God a chance and just come!

PROMISE 5

Galatians 3:13 "Christ has redeemed us from the curse of the law, having become a curse for us, for it is written, cursed is anyone who hangs on a tree."

If you know the story of Adam and Eve, you know they sold out to the devil. The earth and its inhabitants were under the care of Adam. God made just one demand on Adam and his wife, Eve. God told Adam that he could eat of all the trees of the garden except the one called the tree of the Knowledge of Good and Evil, because the day that they would eat from it, they would die. God had made every tree that was pleasant and good for food. They had no reason to disobey and therefore sin, but they did. This act of grave disobedience and sin cost greatly. Their eyes were open to see as God sees. Sin entered into the world and was bred into humanity.

Once this happened, God *had* to put them out of the beautiful garden. You see, He had also planted another tree in the midst of the garden called the Tree of Life. God, of course, knew that if either of them ate from the Tree of Life, our sin nature would live forever. And since sin separates us from the presence of God, this would have meant that we would have had to spend eternity separated from God. How heartbreaking for God to be separated from all mankind. But Adam and Eve gave in to satan, and he became the ruler of this world. Now they would have to live under his dominion. Under his dominion came laws and a curse over the world and mankind.

You can find the laws listed in Deuteronomy 28. This is not a comprehensive list, either. The curse is extreme. The good news is that God made a way for anyone who chooses to come back into fellowship with Him. Christ came to earth to redeem us, to buy us back, and to free us from the curse.

What does all of this have to do with being overweight? Everything that is bad and evil is part of that curse. Being overweight causes pain, sickness, and heartache—none of which God ever intended.

When Christ bought us back with His life, the curse was broken over us. We now have the right to live free of any kind of pain, sickness, disease, or emotional stress.

If you have ever been fat, you can attest to the emotional pain a fat person goes through. It can be sheer torment at times. Thank God, we have a choice to receive the "get out of fat free" card because of Jesus Christ. He paid our debt, and He did it because He loves us. His life was the high price of our bondage to food or anything else that tries to keep us from the life God has for us. We now have total freedom. You can receive it now. You've been bound too long! Be loosed in Jesus' name.

God's offer of salvation is extended to anyone and everyone. Still, He leaves the decision up to the individual. He created us to think for ourselves and make our own decision. We have the right to make wrong choices.

God will protect your rights, whether you're making the proper choice or not. However, don't dismiss the consequences to every decision made. Your right to suffer will be adhered to.

The smartest thing we can do is to get on God's side and stay there. It is true that we do not have to work for our salvation—it's a free gift from God, and Jesus died for us to be set free. We do, however, need to work very diligently to maintain closeness with our Father.

It's up to us, individually, to get acquainted with God and the Bible. We need to know Him better than we know ourselves. After we get to know Him, we are told to imitate Him. How great is that? We are to act like God, do what He does, say what He says and expect what he expects!

PROMISE 6

Gen 1:26(a) "Let Us make man in our image."

The Bible tells us that God made man in the very image of Christ and God. It would seem that we started out in pretty good form. *So what happened?*

I know in my case, my parents trained me to eat wrong and to live an unhealthy lifestyle. That's all I knew when I was growing up. I either had too little or too much.

We were never taught to find that place of balance. Then, of course, with all the bad training, it set me up for a lifetime of misery. It has been a difficult thing to grow up with a deficit from childhood. I have always tried to be normal, whatever that was. I just knew that I didn't look like the other kids, and my heart was breaking all the time.

I was being abused throughout my life by many people, some who didn't even know me. A bombarding of very unkind words and put-downs, for a child can be devastating. Abuse leaves scares no matter how it comes.

You may be thinking, "Come on! Not *everyone* treated you badly." It seemed like it to me. I was treated differently than the others throughout my childhood and teen years. Today we would call it discrimination. If you haven't noticed, we live in a very unforgiving world. It doesn't really matter if it's your fault or not, you will be the one to pay the price of the stigma society places on the obese.

My plea to parents is, don't let this happen to your children. You might not like what I'm about to say, but letting your children overeat and become overweight is a form of child abuse. I can't stress it enough, please don't allow it. Use every means available to you to see that your child doesn't grow up like I did. Your children are your responsibility, and their future is in your hands. You can't expect someone else will deal with it. You're the parent.

PROMISE 7

I John 4:4 "You are of God, little children, and have overcome them, because He, who is in you, is greater than he who is in the world."

I want you to succeed in all that you do, and I believe Christ really is the answer. Why do I believe that? I can't begin to tell you of all the real miracles I have seen in my own family. I knew it was God who had worked these miracles, and I know He still does miracles today. We have witnessed miraculous things through the challenges of brain tumor, colon cancer, lupus, alcoholism, and more. Some folks will never be convinced, but as for me, I don't need to be convinced. I know for a fact that God is real, and He is a good God! I also know that He is no respecter of persons. God loves you as much as He loves me and my family. He wants to help you in all that you do in life, even weight issues.

With God's help, I have overcome obesity in my life. Do I need to watch what I eat? Sure I do, if I want to remain healthy and look good. I also need to brush my teeth if I don't want cavities. There are just some things that we need to get into the habit of doing. Being as wise as we possibly can is a good habit to have. God says in His Word, "My people are destroyed for a lack of knowledge" (Hosea 4:6). The knowledge is out there, we just need to set our minds to find it. God tells us to ask, seek, and knock, and doors will be open for us. We have a big part in getting wisdom for life's issues. We need to know how to live longer and keep our kids living longer. Eating better is very important.

I must tell you, though: someone can have all the knowledge in the world and still fail because they might not have wisdom. A person could read, study and pump themselves full of good stuff, but if they don't know how to put all that knowledge to work for them, it will be useless. Have you found that out yet? This has nothing to do with you being a Christian or not. It's just a fact.

Many of us could write volumes on how to lose weight, but if we don't put our knowledge to work, what good is it? But you and I can be overcomers. How do I know? God said so!

PROMISE 8

Romans 8:37 b "Yet in all things, we are more than conquerors through Him who loved us."

God wants us to prosper and be in health. He wants us to be victorious and not become a victim of satan. Jesus came to give us abundant life. Sickness, disease, or lack in any area of life, in my opinion, is not living in abundance. John 10:10 says, "The thief does not come except to steal, kill, and destroy. I have come that they may have life, and that they have it more abundantly." This is Jesus speaking. The thief is the devil.

He has given each one of us everything that it will take to conquer all that is set before us. This would include the enemy's ploy to destroy our health, emotional well-being, and our high standard of life that God planned for us.

The problem is, many people don't know it and maybe, never will. Some people think it is God's will for them to be sick. If it's God's will, they wouldn't go to the doctor or take medicine, as not to go against God's will. They wouldn't be trying to get better would they? It's the lack of knowledge that keeps them thinking like that. The knowledge is offered through the Word of God, the Bible. It's up to each individually to read it and believe or reject it. If you are a parent, it's your responsibility to teach your children, and like it or not, you will be held accountable before God with what you chose to teach them. You can teach them to receive all that God has for them or let them, perhaps, suffer lack all their lives.

According to the Bible, we are kings and priests of the Lord. I think it's time we took back our stuff from the devil! God's Word makes it plain just how we are to do that. We are to imitate God in all His ways and speech. If God said it, we need to say it. If God tells us in His Word that we have authority over the devil and the demons, I say we do.

We need to find in God's Word where He tells us to take the authority, and we need to say these scriptures with confidence. I John 5:14-15 says, "Now this is the confidence that we have in Him, that if we ask anything according to His will, He hears us, And if we know that He hears us, whatever we ask, we know that we have the petitions that we have asked of Him."

Look in Matthew 18:18, where Jesus says, "Assuredly, I say to you, whatever you bind on earth will be bound in heaven, and whatever you loose on earth will be loosed in heaven." Do you know what that means? It means you have authority to lock out the enemy or bind him-meaning to tie him up. This means you can release the power of God and order the devil and his demons to be gone, in the name of Jesus!

Please do not try to attempt this in your own power or in your own name; it will not work. Without God, you have no power.

Look at Matthew 16:19, "And I will give you the keys of the kingdom of heaven, and whatever you bind on earth will be bound in heaven, and whatever you loose on earth will be loosed in heaven." See how Jesus uses the example of keys with the power to lock and unlock things, to bind and to lose? Keys represent authority. If you give someone the keys to your home, you have given them the authority to unlock your home and enter it. When you take your keys back, you take back their authority to enter your home. They are bound out of your house, or, you could say, "locked out."

God has given us the keys to everything we will ever need here on earth. The keys that lock and unlock these things are His Word, the Bible. Do you now see the importance of knowing the Word of God? It is literally your weapon against the enemies of this world. Use the keys to become more than a conqueror through Christ.

PROMISE 9

Ps. 103:1–5 "Bless the Lord, O my soul: And all that is within me bless His holy name! Bless the Lord, O my soul, And forget not all His benefits: Who forgives all your iniquities, Who heals all your diseases, Who redeems your life from destruction, Who crowns you with loving-kindness and tender mercies, Who satisfies your mouth with good things, So that your youth is renewed like the eagle's."

We are promised many benefits in this passage, all of which we can use in our quest to lose weight, once and for all.

You are blessed, you are forgiven, you are redeemed, you are satisfied, and your youth is renewed. How great is that?!

I want you to notice something here. David is talking to himself. He is making a demand of himself to say the promises of God. Say them out loud to your own self and let yourself hear the Word spoken.

Let God's Word go down inside of your heart and grow. This is so very important for us to understand. It is the spoken Word of the Lord that works for us and in us. This is the why we need to speak the Word of God aloud. Let the devil hear it, let God's angels hear it, and let yourself hear it.

Ps. 103:20-21 says, "Bless the Lord you His angels, Who excel in strength, who do His word, heeding the voice of His word. Bless the Lord, all you His hosts, You ministers of His, who do His pleasure." Wow! When the Word of God is spoken with our voice, the angels are commanded to do the will of God.

Psalm 91:16 says, "With long life I will satisfy him, and show him My salvation." You and I are promised a long and satisfying life.

Ecclesiastes 7:8a, says that the end of a thing is better than the beginning. You can end up better than when you started. That's the goodness of God.

So, are you satisfied yet? If not, keep going and keep finding out more of the will of God for your life, get in it, and live life.

Read all of Psalm 91. It is filled with good things that the Lord wants us to have. Take a close look at 91:1–2. These two verses are extremely important because it's an, "I will if you will" scripture. If you will "dwell in the secret place of the Most High and abide under the shadow of the Almighty and say of the Lord, "He is my refuge and my fortress; my God, in Him I will trust," then you can count on reaping the harvest that God promises in the rest of the chapter. Only then can you receive the protection and promises of God.

The only way you and I can receive the salvation of God is to receive Jesus Christ as our Lord and Savior. Having the help of the Lord is so wonderful. I no longer am trying to do things on my own and in my own strength. You can receive the gift of Christ right now, and all that comes with it. It's the gift of freedom from a life of being tired, overweight, sick, and depressed. But remember, a gift has to be received before it can be enjoyed.

When you are reading these scriptures, don't forget the rule. God says, "I will, if you will." You'll find that most of these scriptures have a condition to be met. I truly believe the biggest reason we don't see more answers to our prayers is that we just don't take the time and effort to meet God's simple conditions. The Bible says in James 4:2–3, "You lust and do not have. You murder and covet and cannot obtain. You fight and war. Yet you do not have because you do not ask. You ask and do not receive, because you ask amiss, that you may spend it on your pleasures."

Remember when I said that I prayed to the Lord that He would either make me thin or kill me? Can you see how I prayed amiss? If I would have known better, I would have prayed like this: "Lord, I can't do this by myself. I need Your help. I need Your wisdom on how to lose weight. I believe that you hear me and will answer me, in Jesus' name."

It definitely was not God's will to kill me. I wanted to die, but He wanted me to live life to the fullest. As a child, I cried out for help many times but no one close to me knew what to do, no one had the wisdom of God and no one knew Christ.

As I look back, I remember there were many missed opportunities for us to know God on a personal level. I remember my parents sending us to church at Christmas time because they gave away fruit and nut baskets. They could have taken us and perhaps gotten saved way back then. Our lives would have been so different.

Some might be saying, "I am a Christian and I am fat, even obese. Why aren't things changing for me?" Check your heart for the answer. What's going on in your life? Not all, but most overweight people eat too much and eat the wrong things. Be honest with yourself, is that you? I'm not judging you in any way, but if you are reading this book, I will assume that you want to lose weight and get healthy. Or maybe it's your child or another family member that needs help.

Honesty is the key here, but if you, or they, keep lying to yourselves/themselves, you will never make the changes that need to be made. The problem needs to be out in the open so that it can be fixed.

I am not a psychologist, just someone who has been through it all and came out on the other side. I know the tricks, lies, and deceptions that go on in the minds of the obese, and the pain and disgust that comes with being fat. The uncontrollable desire to eat everything in sight and still be hungry was never ending. I know how it feels to have hunger pains at night that keep you awake, and the tears, even as an adult that are shed many nights.

I know the feeling of wanting to run away where no one knows you or cares about you. I know the pain of trying to dress for an occasion and emptying out your entire closet and still finding nothing but the baggy shirt and super-size pants that look horrid, but it's all that fits. I know the hurt of the stares and comments of heartless people, including children. I get it! I truly know.

တ

~ 42 ~

Be The Parent

When you read about my school days, know that what I wrote was just minimal to the challenges I went through as an obese student. This is why I want so badly for moms and dads to read and act on the advice given. Yes, your child may feel unloved and unsatisfied when you say, "No, you can't have that," or "come on, we are walking for twenty minutes," but, trust me, they'll live, and they will get over it.

You will become the hero! When prom night gets here and she is wearing the outrageously gorgeous size six gown, you'll shine with pride in her, and in yourself for helping her achieve a life of health, and of course beauty. She will never forget you for saying no to overeating at a young age as she looks in the mirror and sees God's beautiful young lady looking back.

Don't forget the son on his wedding day admiring himself in the mirror just before he marries the love of his life. He stands tall and well built. Not an inch of fat and not one bad memory of being hounded in school with the fat jokes and ridicules. Thanks to you, he is a proud young man that will pass the good eating habits along to your grandchildren.

There is another side to the outcome of a parent who lets their child eat whatever and whenever they want. Nine times out of ten, you won't even hear about the prom until it's over. There will be no dates, no good memories, and no long-lasting friendships. You'll have the kid that makes everyone laugh, the clown that is the butt of the good times for others. He never has a date and ends up angry at the world. Believe it or not, if you listen close through his bedroom door in the middle of the night, you will hear the tears of the clown.

You might have the daughter who eats to soothe the pain of not going on the ski trips with friends because if she fell down, she wouldn't be able to get back up. Maybe she's not going on the field trips because the accommodations didn't account for her size. The beach party? Forget it. She has already heard all the whale jokes. Even though she tells you that it doesn't matter, it hurts like heck, and no one is the wiser. She turns to food as her friend and comforter. Her life just gets worse and more lonely. By this time, it takes more food to do the comforting job right.

You see where this is going, right? You can change history right now for your kids, if you are willing. You can use your authority to save a life from the pain and embarrassment of obesity. I know parents today want to be their kids' friend. You know, they probably have a lot of really cool friends, but only one mom and dad, just be their parents.

൜

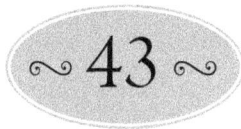

～43～

Did You Know?

- Did you know that childhood obesity and Diabetes are the number one diseases in children?

- Did you know that your children will, "Do as you do, not as you say?"

- Did you know that childhood obesity has tripled in the past few decades?

- Did you know that cruelty doesn't discriminate? It will go for a child or adult.

- Did you know that an upright man can never be a downright failure?

- Did you know that strength is attained by meeting resistance?

- Did you know that if you worry there is no need to pray, and if you pray there is no need to worry?

- Did you know that eating real butter is better for you than margarine?

- Did you know the best thing you can spend on your children is time?

- Did you know that the time to make friends is before you need them?

- Did you know that you can either make or break a habit in twenty one days?

- Did you know that weight charts were made by skinny people?

- Did you know that eating too few calories will stop your weight loss?

- Did you know that a calorie is a calorie no matter how you eat it?

- Did you know that you can have your cake and eat it too?

- Did you know that it's what you learn after you know it all that counts?

- Did you know that children may tear up the house, but they seldom break up the home?

- Did you know that salmon is better for you than tuna?

- Did you know that Orange Roughy doesn't taste fishy?

- Did you know that lobster is the cockroach of the sea?

- Did you know that there are high concentrations of pesticide residues in raisins and peanuts?

- Did you know that you should always eat breakfast? It jump starts your metabolism.

- Did you know that your reality check just might clear?

- Did you know that the odds of a piece of bread landing jelly side down are 50/50?

- Did you know that proper response to 'Good Morning' is not 'Prove it?'

- Did you know that life is a piece of cake but I'm still on a diet?

- Did you know that many are called but very few return their messages?

- Did you know that you should drink lots of water but not from your faucet?

- Did you know that you can get used to 2% milk?

- Did you know that you can use applesauce instead of oil when making a cake?

- Did you know that "I Can't believe it's Not Butter" spray has no calories or fat and tastes great?

- Did you know that fat-free whipped cream is great in coffee?

- Did you know that you should eat live things to live longer?

- Did you know that God loves you?

- Did you know that He created you and has a plan for your life?

- Did you know that you can do all things through Christ who strengthen you, even losing weight?

- Did you know that God is waiting to hear from you?

- Did you know His phone number is Jeremiah 33:3?

- Did you know that if anything is going to change, you need to change it?

- Did you know the grass is greener on the other side because someone's watering it?

- Did you know your story isn't over yet? Just turn the page!

- Did you know life can change with one word from the Lord?

- Did you know He needs your permission to speak that one word?

- Did you know that your future is in your mouth?

- Did you know you can take your life back?

୭

❧ 44 ❧

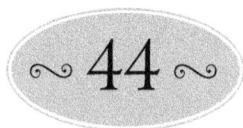

You Can Do This

Sometimes life can get real tough. Sometimes you might think that you just can't go on.

The world we live in today is so full of bad and hurtful things. Stop adding to your hurt by being down on yourself. What good is that going to do? There is a way that will help us to live a better life. Jesus said "I am the way, the truth and the life. No one comes to the Father except through Me." He's even so much more than that. He is our peace that passes all understanding.

In this world today, peace is a commodity. It seems to me that something comes along nearly every day to try and steel that peace from us. That very same thief will do it's best to steal our children's peace as well. Being an overweight or obese child or teen can cause such devastating, emotional and physical distress, that it would become nearly impossible to hold on to a peaceful life without God.

The crazy thing is, even some people who have received Christ as their Savior, are living without the fulfillment of many of the promises of God in their lives, because they don't even know they are available to them. Even though God and Jesus has made things like peace available to everyone, not everyone will receive it. The ones that will ask, seek, knock, are the ones that will find what they need to live life to the fullest. *Just something to think about.* If God is willing and able to make the lives of our children and that of ourselves better, what holds us back from receiving Him and His love?

❧

~ 45 ~

No Magic—Just God

It's been years since I began my search for the magic bullet or pill or whatever would make me skinny. Like I said before, they all work to a point. That point being the birthday party, the barbeque, the vacation, or whatever else might come up. I find that for me, it all boils down to my flesh. I either kill the flesh or feed it. I realized that I can't have it both ways.

When I made up my mind that I couldn't live my life overweight and miserable, I surrendered to a life of eating better food to have a healthy, nice-looking body.

For some, that may not be the goal. For me, I needed to not only feel good but I needed to look good in my own eyes. Do I miss the ice cream, cake, and snickers? YES! But I look good. When I look good, I feel good inside and I function much better. Don't get me wrong, I'm not a bean pole, but I'm not obese or overweight anymore. I die daily to my fleshly desires. Now, I say when and what I eat, not my demanding flesh.

~

~ 46 ~

The Flesh Needs To Die!

I needed to have a funeral and invite Ben & Jerry and the whole McDonald's gang. "Oh Henry, you, and Mr. Good Bar are invited too. Sarah Lee and Marie Calendar are coming with Mrs. Fields. What an impact you have all made in this life!"

"Dearly beloved, we are gathered here today to say goodbye to someone you were all very close to. She spent so much time with all of you "fattening indulgencies." I know it will be very hard for you to let her go. You'll just have to get used to not seeing the big smile on her face when she saw each of you.

How she loved you all! She was so dedicated to you; so loyal. Her heart jumped for joy at the very sight of every one of you. She might have even died for you, but towards the end something happened.

You see, years ago she asked Jesus to come into her heart and save her, and He did. He saved her spirit and His Word renewed her mind, but her flesh went wild, until now. Today she found out that the Word of God says in Romans 8:13 that if she lives according to the flesh she will die, but if by the Spirit, she will put to death the deeds of the body, the flesh...she will live!

So from this day forth she will not walk according to the flesh but according to the Spirit. Her flesh has been put to death by the Spirit of the Living God. Because of this, none of you will be able to torment her ever again. You are dismissed."

Maybe you need to have your own funeral and plan a guest list. Just bury the things that have stopped you from living the life that God has planned for you. Satan would love to keep you bound by the deception that "you can't." Well, I'm here to tell you that you can and you will.

It won't be easy, and it will take a lifetime of being on guard. Satan comes to steal, kill, and destroy, but God came to give us life, and that more abundantly. Good for us. (John 10:10)

If you're a parent and you're asking what you can do for your overweight child, here's the answer. Stop being their friend and be the parent. Don't ask them what they want. Give them what they need to grow up to be healthy and live long.

Your child doesn't need another playmate, they need someone to love them enough to lead them and guide them in the right things of life. Do you want your kids to outlive you? Then do the right things for them. Help them to make the right choices. You can do this. If you can't do it alone, get some help, but do it. Save your child's life and stop them from being me.

Don't ever give up. I am fifty nine years old and I can't tell you the times that I just wanted to roll over and give up, but I just refused to give in and let the devil win. I have too many things to do and I will run my race and I will finish my course. It will be when God and I decide I'm finished, not the devil!

∽

～ 47 ～

You Can Overcome Anything!

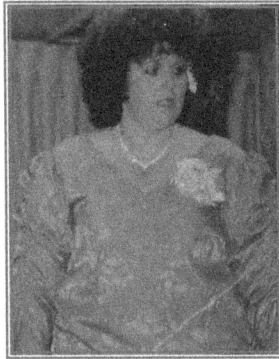

I'm not where I want to be yet, but I'm not where I was. Thank You, Lord. The heartbreaking thing is, I didn't have to go through any of this. I could have had a more normal childhood, adolescent years, and teens if my parents would have known better. Parents, in this day and age we really have no excuse.

The information is out there if you want it. I hear excuses all the time why parents won't do this. "It's too hard, too expensive, and too time consuming." What you're saying then is that your kids are not worth it. You're too busy to do the right things to help them grow up with self-esteem, and confidence.

My parents could have gotten the information that would have changed my life. They were too busy to notice what I was going through. Please do not make that mistake with you or your children. It is so unnecessary.

I don't know anyone who doesn't have access to a computer and internet. Every library has this service available to you. Everyone has access to a doctor or health care provider. I also believe that the Lord has given us a knowing from right and wrong, even when it comes to eating. If God made it, eat it, and if man made it, don't eat it. How's that sound? It's a good start.

Our kids need to be encouraged to play outside. They are lacking exercise and fresh air. The world has taken from our children the pleasures of outdoors and turned them into 'indoor game junkies.' Parents, you're the boss. You're the teacher; you're the last word on everything in your child's life.

ᕙᕗ

~ 48 ~

Does It Cost More To Eat Right?

Now let's talk about this myth of it costing more to eat right than to eat badly. I've heard this most of my adult life and I bought into it. We need to find out the truth and not just assume others are right. If you're willing to put a little time into it, you will be surprised at what you find.

In this chapter we'll learn better choices that you can make for your family that will be good, and inexpensive. You don't have to eat Macaroni and Cheese all the time just because you think it's cheaper than the good stuff.

To start with, I don't know of one person who will sit down and have one serving of Mac and Cheese. Do you actually know how much one serving is? One serving of a 7.5 oz. box of Mac and Cheese is 2.5 oz. which isn't even one cup. If you have very small children you might get away with one cup each but if you're serving kids five and older, one cup will not fill them up.

The direction tells us to add a fourth of a cup of milk, and four Tbsp. of butter or margarine. The calories per serving prepared are 410, remember that's for less than one cup. Most kids 5 and older will consume 1.5–2 cups per meal. (Older kids will consume most of the box.) That would be 615–820 calories per meal. The cost of the meal for 3 servings= around $2.50 (including ingredients). If you are serving 3 kids you will need 2 boxes which = $5.00 to make. Older kids will eat more therefore the cost will be more. Plus, in about an hour, they will be hungry again because you fed them all carbs. Carbohydrates will never fill you up, and only satisfy for a short period of time. Let's just say you gave them an apple with the meal, (added cost) this will help with the quick onset of hunger that is sure to come.

Now, let's try something different. What if instead of Mac and Cheese, you used a box of whole grain Linguine (13.25 oz.) There are 7 servings in the box. The whole box cost about $2.20. Open a large can of tomato sauce and add to it some oregano, Italian spice, a little sugar, a little salt, and some garlic. Simmer while the pasta is cooking and put it over the pasta, add a few crackers or a piece of whole wheat bread and you have a better meal that will feed many.

The whole grain pasta is a good source of fiber and the tomato sauce in a good source of vitamin C, A, K, potassium, magnesium, fiber, chromium, B-1, B-6, foliate, iron, B-5, vitamin E, and Lycopene. These are just a few of the benefits of the tomato and they are only about 30–35 calories each.

Anyone can come up with a more nutritious meal that won't break the bank if they'll get creative. Do it for your family, do it for yourself. There are discount super stores that are a great place to shop for a bargain. The farmers market is an inexpensive place to buy fruits and vegetable and most every town have a couple of them. If you have friends with fruit trees, don't be shy; ask if you can pick some. Most people never use it all and it goes to waste.

I suggest that you can make a big pot of homemade soup that will last for a couple of days and won't cost much, season it well and use free range chicken broth. The broth is a couple of dollars and don't forget to use your coupons. You can also use Braggs Amino; available at most stores. You can add a box of onion soup mix for more taste.

I know some people have a thing about eating the same thing two days in a row. So, on the second night make a Sheppard pie out of the left over soup. You can also make little pot pies for each person. You can add meat if you want too. Make a green salad and a dish of celery sticks with peanut butter or garlic cream cheese, homemade of course.

Many people think fish is too expensive, but it really isn't. You can buy one serving packs of Salmon, Tilapia, and others for only 99 cents each. For a family of five that's less than $5.00. Make some homemade fries and green beans and you're good to go. If they need dessert, don't forget the popcorn. It's also fun to make flavored popcorn.

Have breakfast for dinner, it's cheap and tastes good as well. Don't believe all you hear about eggs, they're really good for you and inexpensive. I find that chicken is most always an inexpensive choice. Look for the brands that don't inject their products with hormones or steroids. Buy the chicken breast with the bone in and take it out yourself. The price difference is amazing. You can do so much with chicken, and eat for less.

Try buying canned salmon at discount markets, it easily feeds four people and it tastes great. If you have left over chicken, make chicken strips the next day for lunch. You can also make Chicken salad with mayo, mustard, grapes, and add walnuts if you have them on hand.

Don't forget about a big pot of beans with cornbread, it doesn't cost much, and most people like it. Beans are a great source of protein and fiber and if you have any left over, make refried bean burritos for lunch the next day or for dinner. Add a salad and some fruit and you did it again. You made a great, good-for-you meal for very little. You don't need a five-course meal every night; a couple of things are ok. (Too much food is one reason I got so fat.) Sometimes a baked potato topped with broccoli, a little shredded cheese and a salad will do.

If you train the kids early to adapt to what you serve, you won't have a problem with complaints. I know dessert is important to most, and you can find many good recipes on the internet, like peanut butter no-bake cookies. You can make Jell-O and put in fresh fruit and a few marshmallows, add nuts if you like them. A baked apple with a small scoop of frozen yogurt is a great sweet treat. Sweet potato pie is good if you use a lot of spices and sugar substitute, no aspartame. Homemade caramel popcorn is always a great treat and a lot goes a long ways.

৵

～ 49 ～

Train Them Up In The Way They Should Go

We all need to understand how important it is to train our kids at a young age, in every area of life. The Bible assures us that if we will train them young, when they are older, they won't depart from that training. On the other hand, with wrong training, they could grow up with bad habits that could actually cause great harm and even an early death. No parent would want that, yet we are guilty of teaching them wrong in the name of love. Like I said before, my parents thought they were showing me love by feeding me so much. What they were actually doing was reinforcing bad habits in me. They were setting me up for failure. The thing is, when this happens, we most likely will pass these mistakes, unknowingly, to our children unless we become knowledgeable and make needed changes. Here we see the generational curse begin making its way down the line, generation after generation, unless someone stops it.

Generational curses are judgments passed on to the next generation. Overeating, gluttony, and bad habits are generally something passed down from our parents and grandparents.

Satan doesn't play by the rules. He will use any means to steal, kill and destroy; he'll even use food. The beauty of it is, you as a parent, can stop him dead. You have more power and control of your child's life than anyone on this planet.

The Bible tells us that if we have given our lives to Christ, we have the same power and authority as Jesus does, and that's a lot of power. We then have the right to back satan off of our kids and out of our homes.

We, as parents, have to protect our kids from the evil that lurks everywhere. This world has gone astray and is trying to steal a generation of children from their health and life.

Look at the ads on television, especially during the cartoons. They have become a training ground for over-indulgence and reinforcement of bad habits. Notice how many commercials are about bad food, bad drinks, and a lack of self-control. They show kids having the biggest drink, the biggest hamburger with the biggest fries, and let us not forget the biggest ice cream, cake, candy, and cookies. When a kid pours a bowl of cereal, it's a serving for three. You get my point.

It's our job to be there to explain the difference between one serving and three. If we, as parents, don't know the difference, we have a problem. My grandson was doing this until I showed him the box with the serving size listed and the calorie intake. Now he pays closer attention to the serving size and eats accordingly.

We need to monitor the eating habits of our children as well as to teach them right from wrong. Some may think it's a waste of time to be saying this because every parent should just know it. My parents didn't know it. I didn't realize it myself until I was trying to find out how to lose my excess weight. You can go a lifetime and not know or understand if no one tells you.

If you are reading this book, you now know, and are responsible for what you do with the information you have learned. I want to encourage you not to just close the book and do nothing. The Bible tells us, to know the right things to do and not do it is sin, (my interpretation) (James 4:17). Besides, don't you want the best for your family and yourself? Of course you do. Do your own research and don't just take my word for it. Then you will have no doubts.

෴

∼ 50 ∼

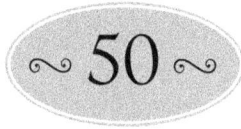

Never Too Late

It's never too late to change and make a difference. Your children have a lifetime ahead of them. You have it in your power to do all you can to make it a life worth living. If you make the right decisions now, they won't be spending needless time trying to figure it out later. They'll have enough the deal with.

You are your child's hope for a life of healthy habits and good choices. You can be a part of fixing any eating problems that they may be having. Remember, you're not alone. There is help. Sometimes it may seem you'll never find it, but you will, because you want too. You are showing them your love by helping them find answers.

Love is not another box of cookies. Love sometimes has to say no. Love sometimes has to walk with your kids when you don't feel like it. Love takes them to the park instead of sending them to their room with a video game for hours. Loves gets them to the doctor for help, and if that doctor doesn't help, find another one and another one until someone gets it.

∼

∾ 51 ∾

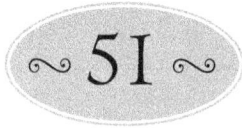

What About You?

Let's talk about you as the parent, caretaker, or guardian. Are you the best you can be, or have you let your guard down concerning your health, eating habits, and weight? I do understand it's a tremendous job of having the responsibility of raising children, and some are now raising the grandkids. You are to be commended and praised, and I, in no way, want to diminish the enormous challenge of raising kids.

This I know: you need to take care of yourself, first. If you can receive a better understanding of health and eating right, it will be passed on to the children. On the other hand if you don't get educated on this issue, the family will suffer. You are the leader of the pack and they are looking to you for the answers.

In all reality, the kids are just following the actions of the parents or caregivers. If the head of the household is overweight, we can see where the change needs to come in. If the parent gets retrained, the child will be retrained. Yes, your child might cry and throw a fit, kick, stomp, and scream, but that's ok, let them. You are now in lifesaving mode. Like I said before, they will get over it and thank you later. You can be sure when date night, prom night or wedding night comes, they will truly love you for being the strong parent that you are. The parent that learn to say, 'NO,' to wrong choices.

Take the time and effort to work on you, and the family will follow. I was pretty strict with my daughter as she was growing up. There was no way on the planet I was going to let her become me, and I did say *no*, plenty. She stayed thin until she got married. When she was out from under my care, Cindy and her new hubby, Michael, thought they knew it all and put on a few pounds. Thank the Lord they came to their senses and backed away from over eating. Cindy put on a little weight with the birth of their sons, but most of it came back off. My grandson is nineteen, tall and thin. He works at it and is careful of what he eats, most of the time.

Cindy, my daughter, is a stage-three colon cancer survivor. She was diagnosed with cancer when she was in her early thirties. The new chemotherapy killed the cancer cells but did something weird to her body. She got really thin at the time she was undergoing the chemo, but when it was stopped, she gained a lot of weight in places where she had been thin before chemo. This was devastating to her. She is a tiny person with a small frame. Through the years, she has really worked on losing the extra pounds, and she has, because she never gave up on it.

My younger grandson, Mitchel, struggles with his weight now and then. For him, it comes down to just overeating. He's almost thirteen now and very tall like his dad. We have to constantly reinforce the food facts with him. He exercises with his older brother, when they can, walks with his mom and dad, and they hike and swim in the summer. He sometimes gets upset with us for keeping things under control but he knows it's because we love him. When we made it a family thing to lose or keep the weight off it was easier for him.

I believe having some kind of support system helps a lot with kids. They need to be shown, not just told. As for me, for the first time in my life I am not considered overweight. What an awesome feeling.

Our success is attainable if we don't ever give up. This is also true in every aspect of our lives. Giving up is not an option, ever.

~ 52 ~

Stop The Insanity

You've heard the phrase, "stop the insanity." I think that is such a great idea. We need to just *stop*. Stop worrying about whether we ate too many grapes or the apple we ate was too big. Stop weighing ten times a day thinking something will change. The truth is, it will change. Your weight fluctuates several times a day and most of the time it goes up. Why do we want to torture ourselves like that?

Trust me; that borders on obsession and I used to do that daily. It would only frustrate me and send me into a tailspin, then I wouldn't eat anything the rest of the day, knowing full well that it would send my body into a starve mode.

For me, I weigh in the morning when I get up and forget it. Don't live your day by the scales, live it by good sense. We know we are not going to gain weight by eating a couple of cookies. The problem is that some can't stop after a couple of cookies. It's like the alcoholic trying to have just a couple of drinks. It isn't going to happen. One will lead to many more and a gigantic fall.

It really bothers me a great deal when I hear someone say, "Just eat the cookie, one won't hurt you." Unless you've ever had an addiction, you probably need to keep silent. I don't say this to be disrespectful; you just really don't understand the consequences of such things. It could be a matter of life or death to many. We need to respect people and their wishes and stop trying to push them into something they don't want to do.

~

∾ 53 ∾

Diets

I'd like to share with you some of the things that worked and the things that didn't work for me, and you can research them for yourself.

Each one of us are different and the way we lose weight and maintain our weight will be different. Please do your own research on the things I am about to tell you. I believe in having help to get the job done.

I tried for many years to "just stop eating." Every time I would try to eat normally, more weight would pile on me. Little did I know, when I went on a starvation diet, my body was designed to automatically hold on to the fat because it didn't want to starve. Most of what I ate was stored as fat; it was my body's way of staying alive.

When I would see a weight gain while eating hardly any food, I would become frustrated, give in, and eat everything I could get my hands on. I would start the cycle over, gain more weight, and become depressed and withdrawn. I hated myself even more because I couldn't even go on a stupid diet right. Now, I was worse off than before I started. You probably know just what I mean. What now?

I had to recognize that it was a trap of the enemy to keep me down and out. If he could keep me occupied with weight issues all the time, there would be no time for me to just live life and no time to share the wonderful things God has stored up for my life.

I couldn't see past the fat and I was letting life slide by without living it.

Many of the diets that I have been on were insane. However, some worked to a point. I want to encourage you to do your homework and find what's best for you. In previous chapters I talked about all the stupid diets I've tried, with no success.

In my early days of dieting, I went on Weight-Watchers and I had minimal weight loss. I do, however, know people that have lost weight on this program, but most of them put the weight back on.

I tried some of the pre-packaged diets and did lose a good amount, but it cost me a lot of money; I notice that the celebrities that do their commercials seem to put their weight back on, for the most part.

One of my greatest successes was with a program called *Free to be Thin.* It is a Bible-based program that suggests a support group. Ultimately though, you'll be on your own, so you will need to determine to change your mind and heart about food and weight.

The next successful program I did was Nutra-System. I went on it about twenty years ago, and it was very different than today, so check it out really good before starting. Again, with any program, you need to have a change of mind and heart towards food. Food is not our life.

You can't just go on a diet, lose the weight, and go back to eating the same way. You will put the weight back on quickly. The biggest problem I had with the pre-packaged diet foods was when I started to eat my own food. It didn't taste as good as theirs did, and it was hard to keep the calories down and make it taste good. I couldn't seem to get satisfied. For one year, all my food was premeasured, and I didn't have to think about it. I opened a package, heated it, and ate.

We have to learn about nutrition, portion size, and how to make things taste good, or we will fail once again. It is also very important to learn self-control. After years of indulgence, this was key for me to lose the weight and keep it off. Again, I had to unlearn much and relearn even more.

Although a person can lose weight on the meal-in-the-mail programs, unless you change your thinking and your bad habits, you will regain the weight.

∾

HCG (Human Chorionic Gonadotropin)

The long name is Human Chorionic Gonadotropin. Personally, I have found this to work very well for me. It's very structured and rigid to follow—not hard, just precise. Researchers seem to find no unsafe side effects. (Always check with your doctor before starting a weight-loss program.) It was discovered many years ago by Dr. A.T.W. Simeons. Dr. Simeons researched for many years on obesity, its causes, symptoms and its nature. There is far too much information to list so I suggest you check this one out.

The name of Dr. Simeon's book is, *Pounds & Inches, A New Approach to Obesity.* You can download it on your computer or go to my web site for more information on this: www.youcantakeyourlifeback. org. It's worth investigating. I like the soundness of Dr. Simeon's research findings. I believe Dr. Simeon discovered the answer to obesity years ago.

Many who have followed his protocol have lost weight successfully and have not regained it. I, myself, had such great success with hCG that I became a distributor. I believe in it that much. Most everyone that I have had the pleasure of helping to succeed on this protocol, is very elated with it. I would advise you to do your homework on this and refrain from starting it without being fully informed. Throughout the years, many have changed the original protocol and lessened the quality of the program. Like anything else, money becomes an issue. For best results, you need to acquire the best products. Some HCG products have been cut with various vitamins and other things that actually may weaken the strength of the product. Although vitamins are good for you, you will want to have the purest product you can for best results. My goal is to see everyone who wants to lose weight, succeed. I am available for them through the entire program. This is the most inexpensive program I have ever came across that works. You eat your own food and work on changing your eating habits and metabolism.

On any successful weight-loss protocol, you will need to reevaluate your eating habits and patterns. Remember, if we want change, we will have to change. We cannot keep doing the same thing and expect something different to happen.

To be successful with our weight loss, or that of our children, we need to be informed and have patience. We will also need to be willing to make any changes necessary with the entire family, especially if it's a child that needs to lose the weight.

It's cruel to bake cookies for the family and tell one child he can't have any. The idea is to not make the overweight child feel deprived or left out. We can learn how to satisfy everyone with nutritious foods, even desserts. Check with your pediatrician on the best way to get excess weight off of your child.

I have found that by cutting the empty carbs and sugar nearly clear out of a child's diet, helps them to lose weight very nicely. They can have fruits and vegetables. Stay away from corn and potatoes while they are re-training and trying to lose weight. That means no French fries, not even baked, for now. Have plenty of lean meats, green veggies and all kinds of fruit for dessert. Try making baked apples with cinnamon and a good sugar substitute.

Do your research. You can try Xylitol products or Stevia. Xylitol is a form of sweetener that is said to be good for us. Check out Spry gum and mints. It has been known to guard against cavities because of the Xylitol in it, and my grandson loves it.

✑

Research

My experiences are personal. I have researched and studied weight loss and diet for many years. You can learn a lot from my mistakes, but you still need to research all you can, if you're serious about your weight and that of your family.

Don't leave it up to someone else. No one cares for our children like we do. There is an enormous amount of information on the internet today to help with our battles with weight. Make use of it.

One thing I would suggest is to do plenty of research on the hypothalamus gland. The hypothalamus gland is a huge factor in sustaining weight loss. This gland is in our brain and helps regulate things like hunger, temperature, and sleep. It helps regulate our appetite and sends signals when we are full. This takes about 20 minutes. That tells me that I need to eat slowly to give it plenty of time to work. If your hypothalamus gland is not working properly, you won't get the signal until you have already overeaten, if at all. If it's not working properly, you might be hungry even right after you eat.

There is a way to reset the hypothalamus gland to work for you and not against you. Do the research. You'll be glad you did. Just type in, 'Reset Hypothalamus gland' on a search engine and learn something that could change your life and your family's lives forever.

～ 55 ～

Silence Is Golden

I would like to address those who could possibly have the view that overweight people should just "push away from the table" a little sooner or pray more, read their Bible more, or just have more "willpower." Stop judging overweight people. Unless you are the one struggling with a thing, it's hard to make an educated comment and you certainly cannot stand in the place of judge and jury. Please follow Jesus' actions and have compassion, kindness, and love. Leave the judging to Him if the case warrants it.

I have been judged, ridiculed, and flat out treated badly from well-meaning Christians and family members trying to help me to "get a hold of myself and have a little self-control." Many did not realize that they were close to being my last nerve. I was so close to going over the edge at times; it scared me almost to death, literally. I understand that most people are well-meaning but ignorant on what they are doing to others.

Silence really can be golden at times. Prayer is always the right thing to do for anyone in any situation. Overweight or obese individuals have a hard enough time dealing with the criticism of the rest of the world, let alone from friends and family. It never ceases to amaze me how people actual think they can ridicule and embarrass someone to change. Many in my family tried that approach every chance they had. The only affect it had was that it caused me to sink deeper into a depressed mode. Did they not understand that if I knew how to stop the insanity, I would have done it long ago?

～

～ 56 ～

James 1:5 — Have Wisdom

Speaking to parents, make sure you are not condescending to your overweight child. Ask God for wisdom on how to build them up and not break their spirits. Don't ever allow anyone else to criticize your child, ever. Your job is to protect your child, including from other family members.

Life is so short, we need to live it to the fullest and the healthiest. Help your kids to live long, healthy, happy lives. They will adore, appreciate, and feel protected by you. It's never too late to change things and there is always hope for a good future.

If you need wisdom, ask the Lord for it. James 1:5 tells us that we can have all we want and need just for the asking. What would we do without the wisdom of the Lord?

God made us to be the parent and He has equipped us with the proper tools. Just ask. Our children are the most precious things we have. We need to make sure we take good care of them. To do that, we will need to teach them much about everything we can.

God will help us. He's waiting for us to come to Him, and Jesus has never turned anyone away. He won't start with you or me, trust Him.

You really do hold the future of your children in your hands. You have a chance right now while they are young, to train them and show them the ways of success.

Remember wrong training can be changed in an instant. If you are driving and notice that you went the wrong way, you would immediately stop going that way, turn around and head in the right direction, wouldn't you? It's just that easy to do now in this situation.

Don't delay. Do it today. Change the outcome of their futures.

I know they say that time heals all wounds. I'm not so sure about that, but I am sure that God can. If things don't change, the wounds will remain and possibly be passed on to the next generation to deal with.

I believe it is within our power today to stop this kind of pain altogether. If we, as parents, will wake up and recognize that if we don't take responsibility for what we are able to change, the hurt will go on, tears will flow, the heartache will continue, and our children may die young.

This is not how God intended it to be. I hear people saying that the devil is stealing a generation through video games, rock music, and drugs. Truth be known, it is easier for him to just kill them with food and use their own parents to accomplish it. I know that sounds hard and cold, and sometimes the truth does seem that way. Nevertheless, it still remains the truth.

What's it going to take for all of us to realize obesity is an epidemic and has to be stopped? How many more kids need to grow up to be me? How many will die early because we did not take this seriously? How many children will grow up to be dysfunctional and messed-up when all it would have taken was for someone to say *no*, and to show them a better way. All it would have taken for me, would have been for my parents to pay attention to what was happening and to realize that I was too young to make the right decisions.

Don't let childhood obesity steal your children and grandchildren. Obesity doesn't discriminate, and it's searching for whom it can destroy. Remember, you do have the power to get wisdom to stop the big "O" word in your life, and that of your loved ones. Will you do it?

௸

~ 57 ~

God Really Does Have The Answers

Whether it's losing weight, raising kids, or cleaning your house, God has a correct and successful way of getting the job done. We can keep doing things our way until Jesus comes back, but things will never be right as long as we trust in our own wisdom.

Man's wisdom is so limited compared to the wisdom of God. Can the thing created possibly think it's smarter than the One who created it?

When we begin to search for the answers from the only One with the answers, we have taken our first step towards wisdom. Man has been deceived by the enemy of God into thinking he can handle things on his own.

We were created to depend on our God for everything including the very breath we breathe. Some call it a crutch, others call it fantasy, but the truth remains; without God, we are nothing. Without the Hand of God holding up the universe, we fall into nothingness.

The sooner we realize that no one loves us the way God loves us, the richer our lives will be. Some would say that surrendering to a God that you can't see is being mindless. On the contrary, surrendering to the One who gave us our mind, will and emotions is the smartest, easiest, most wonderful thing anyone can ever do.

God has offered each of us the right to receive His Spirit which is wrapped up in His Son, Jesus. He can live and abide right inside the hearts of mankind. This is an awesome gift from the God who has all power and authority over all things.

∽

∼ 58 ∼

Life Isn't Always Fair

Many things in life doesn't seem fair. Some things seem to be out of order, not going how we planned it, just flat wrong. How is it that many things that happen are not in our best interest? A multitude of things take place in our lives, especially as children, in which we have no control, input or say-so about.

My parents and their lack of knowledge were the main reason I was a fat child. I wasn't sick nor did I have a thyroid problem. I was just fed too much food and trained wrong for a healthy future. My parents were obviously not taught right as children, and that was not their fault either. As an adult, however, I had, and still have, the right and authority to change the things I don't like in my life. What I lacked then was wisdom and know-how.

If we train our children to make right choices when they are young, they will most likely continue with that training into adulthood. Chances are good that they will also pass this training on to their children, thus, we have saved a multitude of generations from obesity. How good is that?

It won't always be perfect, but we can sure do our best to learn and teach. The main thing is to always be willing to get more knowledge and understanding of how God made us to function and what foods work best to keep us alive and well.

❧ 59 ❧

Genetically Altered Food ... Help Or Hindrance?

Genetically altered food could be a real problem for us. I'm not a scientist, but a little common sense can tell us that messing with the plan of the Creator might just be a problem. I've read articles on genetically altered foods, and to be honest, it's scary. Scientists are injecting some of the foods we eat with all kinds of things. It's not just growth hormones and steroids. Also things to keep the bugs away and make the food last longer.

They tell us that too many crops are lost each year because of insect pests. They have come up with a pest spray that will kill the insects alright, but will it kill us, too, over time? Just wondering! Well, that is the part they're not sure of yet. Great!

I read that excessive pesticides and fertilizers can poison the water supply and harm the environment. Let us not forget about the weed killers that are used to protect our altered fruit and veggies. In another article, scientists are saying that they now want to inject our food with different nutrients and vitamins so we won't become deficient. While that may sound very kind and helpful, my question is, what will they take the liberty of injecting next, a birth control of some sort?

I would certainly love to know if all the hormones injected in our meat, poultry and fish isn't partly to blame for the huge rise in obesity.

I heard on the news the other day that by the year two thousand seventeen, seventy five percent of Americans will be considered obese. We need to take the stand of *"not in my family."* Remember, we're going to train up our kids in the way they should go and when they get older they will not be moved by the world's ways. They will already know God's ways and will continue to teach the next generation proper eating habits.

Now, if your kids are already grown, just encourage them to make sure they do all they can to be, and stay healthy. It's never too late to make wise changes.

I've been working on this for years. Even at my age, I am never too old to learn. My plans are to never stop learning. My family, like yours, is so very important to me, and I need them to understand how to live long and strong.

Have you noticed that the doctors today, even with their wonderful educations, seem to know less and less about what's making people sick? There are many new diseases that have them baffled. According to the Bible, it's only going to get worse as time passes.

Obesity, however, can be stopped. Training and re-training is the key. Knowledge is part of the answer, action is the other part. Knowledge without wisdom and action doesn't work. That reminds me of the scripture, "Faith without works is dead." You can have all the faith in the world, but if you never put it to work, it is useless.

My parents knew my being fat wasn't right. They just didn't have the knowledge or the wisdom to know what to do about it. Make it priority to get answers. They assumed it would go away or I would just grow out of it. I didn't grow out of it. I got bigger and bigger and my eating habits got worse.

An unsolved problem just gets bigger. A hurting person just hurts more without a solution, and we all know that hurting people hurt people. I was no exception.

∽

60

Are Fat People Really Happy?

The rumor has it that fat people are happy. Can we just expose that lie right now? I feel that for the most part, fat people are miserable. They can tell me a million times over that they're happy being fat, but I have a very hard time believing it. I was trapped inside of a fat person's body for most of my life and was not a happy person.

I was a great pretender. If people thought I was happy, there wasn't a need for them to feel guilty or sad. Most people don't have a clue of the pain and heartbreak one endures from being overweight or obese. Why would they? Most normal-sized people don't even think about gaining weight or overeating. They don't think about their next meal until they get hungry. Food is not a priority in life, nor is obsessing about how to lose weight.

Most overweight and obese people, including children, just have learned bad habits. If we can learn a bad habit, we can unlearn a bad habit as well. We will need to reverse most of the things that we have learned about food, eating, and what's good or bad. It's not an easy thing to do. It would be so much easier to learn it as a child than to undo it as an adult.

Children, pretty-much do as they are taught. Adults, for the most part, do not like to be told what to do. It's easier to submit when you're a child. Many adults will likely have an attitude of, "I'll do as I please." This makes it a lot harder to deal with life's mistakes that need to be fixed.

I believe anyone can change things, if they have a big enough desire and a will to study, research, and pray. I do understand that many times being overweight is related to a medical condition. If that's the case, a doctor will be your best help. However, the majority of overweight people are that way because of overeating and not enough exercise.

My weapon of choice is walking. I walk almost every day. Do I enjoy it? Not so much, but I do it anyway. The doctors tell me that something as easy as taking a daily walk can add years to your life and help you lose weight and keep it off. Walking strengthens almost everything in you. So, as much as I don't like it, I submit and walk anyway.

When I was at my highest weight, somewhere between 290 and 300-plus pounds (I stopped weighing, so I'm not real sure on the exact number), I did my best to walk as much as one could at that size. As the weight came off, of course, it became easier. It was physically easier, but mentally still very difficult.

I remember walking down the street and having people yell nasty things at me from their car windows. At first, I would cry. I'm sure it was a sight. A thirty-five-year-old fat woman walking down the street, crying. Later, it got to the point where it just didn't hurt anymore. It did not stop me from walking.

I was determined to lose the weight. There were times and seasons where I just really felt like giving up. I had such a long ways to go. Another weapon I had was the one called *never give up attitude.*

The Bible says it like this, "I can do all things through Christ who strengthens me" (Phil. 4:13). So, through the tears and the prayers, I am pleased with my progress.

My hope is that as you read this book, you will acknowledge what I felt and save someone from becoming what I was. Start with your family. Parents, you control what comes in your home. You control the meals that you prepare and the serving sizes.

Make learning to enjoy new foods fun. Insist everyone at least try new things. Find great new ways to cook things. Do it for them. Do it for yourself. Do it for life. I'm proof that this can be done, even at an older age.

Sometimes change is not the easiest thing, but it might be the best thing for you. In my case, and I am sure many of yours, I wanted to change but the right way to get the job done, escaped me.

We all have to take it upon ourselves to search until we find our answers. We have to be determined not to give up, give in, or give out. If we give up, we may never be successful with meeting our goals and desires in life. One thing I now have that I didn't when I was young, is God. I know that with Him, I really can do all things. Christ truly does give us the strength and wisdom needed to be successful in all we set our hearts to do.

Parents, you will need to be strong and stay strong for your children. Don't expect them to think like a grownup. They can't. Think about what you're going to say before you talk with them about anything. When I am reminded of some of the things adults said to me when I was an overweight child, I just have to laugh. Not because it was funny, but because it was insanely dumb. You don't say to a young child, "If you don't like being called fat, lose weight." How crazy is that? You are the adult; help them before they become me.

❦

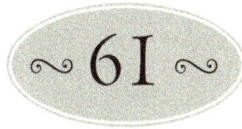

⚭ 61 ⚭

Setbacks

Through the years, I have had many setbacks. Not one of them stopped me from reaching my goal. I refused to give up. We must run our race to the finish. When things get in the way, move them! Remember, you can do all things through Christ who strengthens you. Without Him, not much will ever be accomplished which has lasting effects.

Our life, and the outcome of it, is a choice. It's in our power to change things.

We must remain willing and obedient to be called a winner. Being willing without the obedience part will never get us to the finish line. It's the same with being obedient without being willing. It will only cause us to be stressed out and frustrated with all of life. When we hook the two together, we will have great successes in all life's situations.

⚭

～ 62 ～

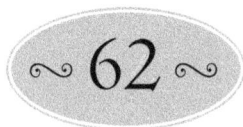

Time To Start Changing

Well, you've made it through the hard truth, the scolding, the praising, and the reality of adult and childhood obesity. I would like to take this time to encourage you to never give up on yourself or your family members. If you're reading this book, you most likely are the one that will be the implementer of change in your household. God has chosen you to retrain and teach the family how to live a long and strong life. What an honor God has placed on you. He trusts you to hear Him and pass on His instructions to your loved ones. You have what it takes and you have the heart's desire to help restore sanity to your family.

My parents loved me very much and I loved them dearly. They did what they knew to do. We didn't have computers, internet, or most of the TV information as we do today. They didn't have access to worldwide knowledge at their fingertips. Knowledge is definitely one of the keys to stop obesity in our families. I know it's possible to get worldly knowledge without God, but as for me, my breakthrough came when I met the giver of all knowledge, Jesus Christ. He holds the keys to life itself, and when we receive Him as our Lord and Savior, He hands us the set of keys to lock and unlock His will for us. We can use the keys or lay them down and forget about them. I chose to use them. You can too.

∽∾

~ 63 ~

Slow And Easy

Start slowly and make simple changes that everyone can do. Sometimes they might not even notice the things you are changing. They will just begin to look and feel better.

You are the prophet of your life and that of your family. Begin to say what you desire, not what you see. Speak to yourself and speak over your family. You will be amazed at what will come about when God's Words come out of your mouth, in faith.

Please do not lay this book down and do nothing. If you need to, read it again and again until it just clicks with you. Your first goal is to start. Do something. Make at least one change today and another one tomorrow. Form new habits that will last generations to come. You can have healthy grandkids before they are even here. If you promote change in your children, you will set in motion what and how they will impart to their children. You can do this!

That's what it's all about. Pay it forward, right?

Our children are the most important people in the world. We can never put them on the bottom of a to-do list. Don't ever let the words, "I love you," remain an unspoken thought. We need to tell them how we feel about them. We need to show them how much we love them by learning the word "*no*" when it needs to be said. We wouldn't let them drink poison, and some foods have the same effect. Say yes to the good stuff. Get them involved in learning how to live a healthy and productive life.

I can't tell you that it will be easy, in fact, it probably won't be easy at all. But I can tell you, it will be the most wonderful, satisfying thing you will ever do for yourself and your family. Have fun and eat to live longer and stronger.

May the Lord give you great wisdom to do this thing called Life, and much compassion for all who cross your path. Stay on God's side—it just works better!

—Lois Peres

❧

A Blessing for You

"The LORD bless you and keep you; The LORD make His face shine upon you, And be gracious to you; The LORD lift up His countenance upon you, And give you peace." Numbers 6:24–26

ം

Prayer of Salvation;

If you have never received Christ as your Savior, do it now. He's waiting for you to come. It will be the easiest, most wonderful thing you will ever do to change your life. Just talk to Him like a friend. He is, you know, and He loves you so very much. If you are like I was, I didn't know how to pray. Someone gave me the words to say, but I really meant them in my heart. I became born again. I prayed something like this:

Lord Jesus, I ask you to come into my heart and be my Savior. I am sorry for the life that I have led. I choose to turn around and go Your way. I renounce the old life style and look forward to a new life in You. I believe in my heart and confess with my mouth, that God raised Jesus from the dead. I receive Jesus as my Lord and Savior. AMEN.

ം

Information Page:

There are many web sites with information on childhood obesity, life style changes, and great recipes for low fat, low calorie cooking. Here are just a few to get you started.

- www.mayoclinic.com/health/childhood-obesity/DS00698

- www.cdc.gov/HealthyYouth/obesity/

- www.foodnetwork.com/shows/index.html

- www.cookingchanneltv.com/

- www.fittv.discovery.com/fansites/blaine/videogallery

- www.delish.com/recipes/best-recipes/low-calorie-recipes

- www.rd.com/healthy-low-calorie-snacks

- www.chiff.com/a/obesity-kids.htm

www.youcantakeyourlifeback.org

or

lois@youcantakeyourlifeback.org

Pictures

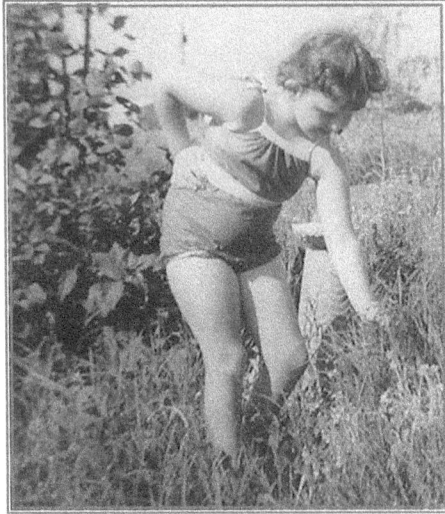

Lois age 4

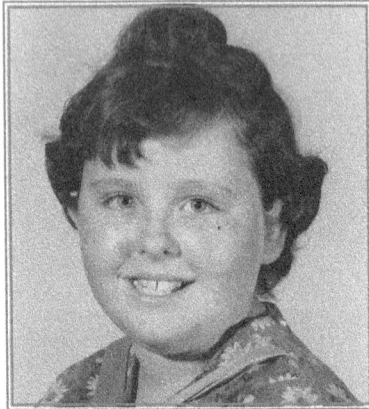

Lois age 9

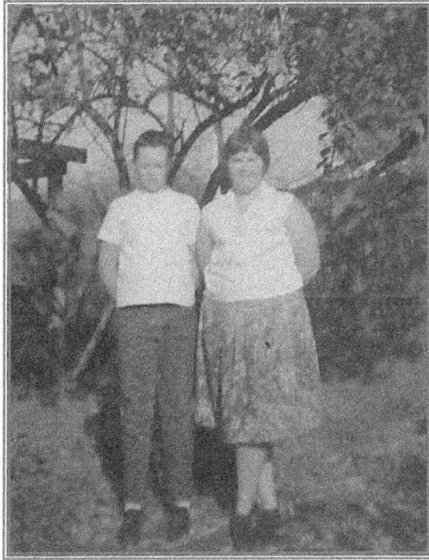

Lois age 13 with her brother

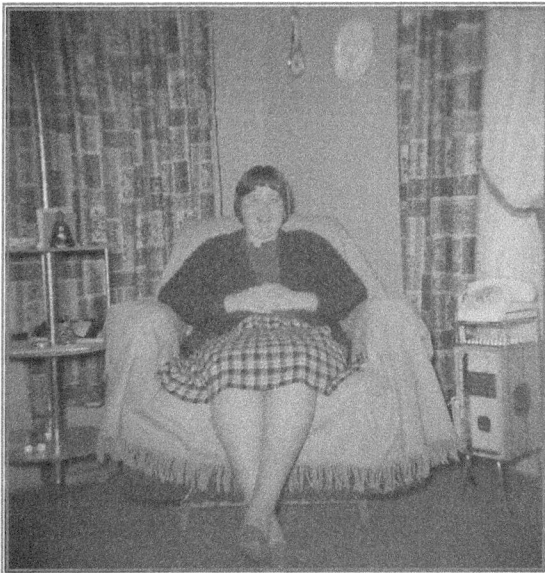

Lois age 13

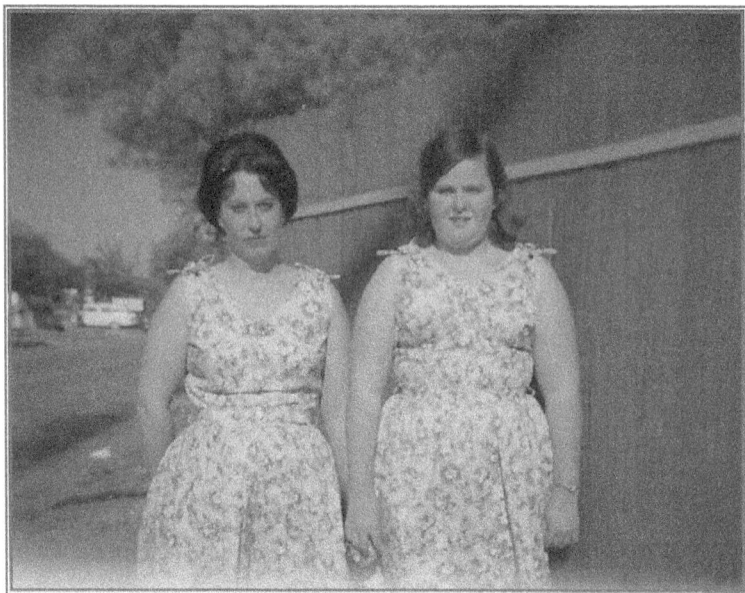

Lois age 14 with her mom

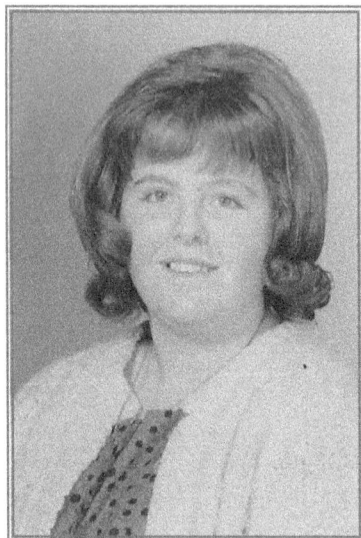

Lois age 15

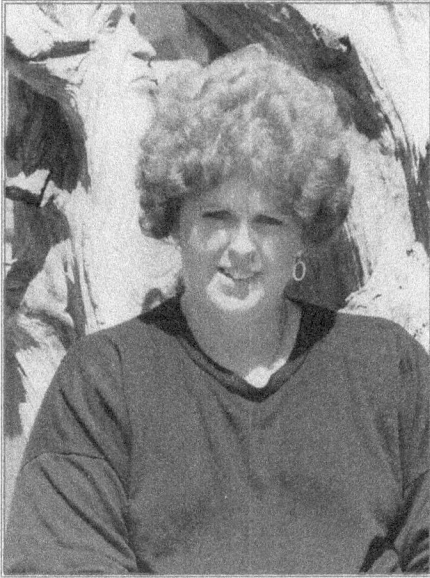

Lois in her 20s

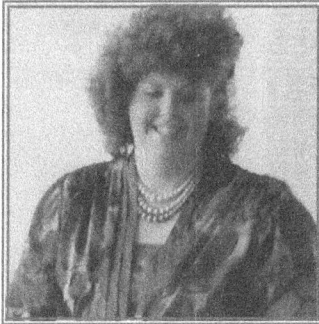

Lois in her 30s

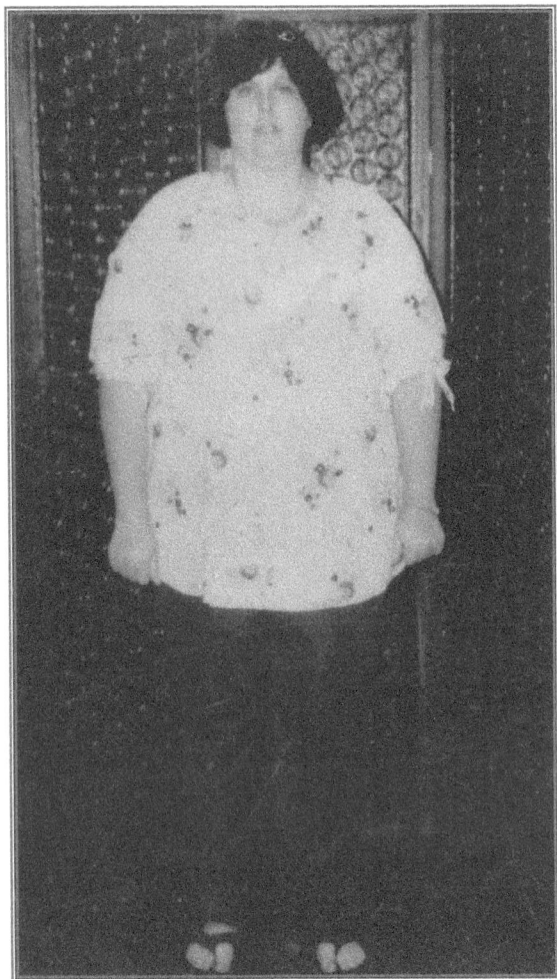

Lois in her late 30s – the diets begin

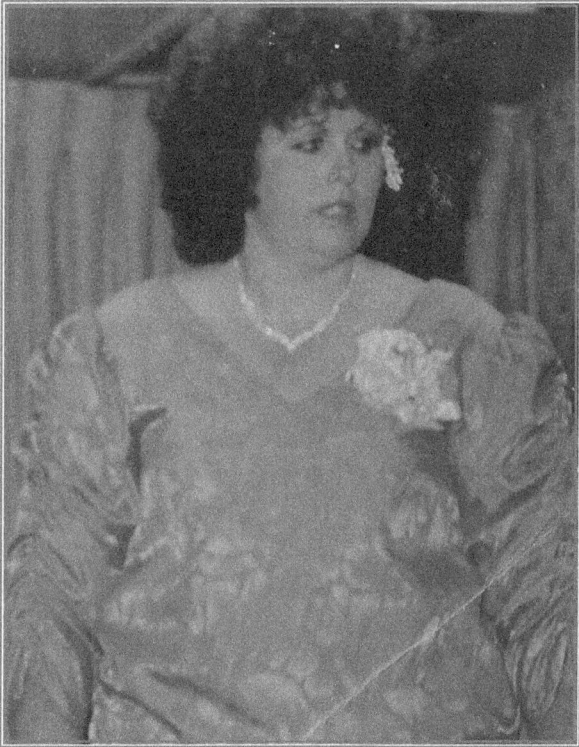

Lois in her early 40s – peak weight 300lbs – "enough is
enough"

www.ingramcontent.com/pod-product-compliance
Lightning Source LLC
Chambersburg PA
CBHW031957040426
42448CB00006B/397